The CROSS *and the* SHROUD

The
CROSS
and the
SHROUD

*A Medical Inquiry
into the Crucifixion*

Revised Edition

FREDERICK T. ZUGIBE

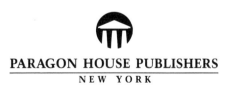

PARAGON HOUSE PUBLISHERS
NEW YORK

REVISED EDITION

Published in the United States by
Paragon House Publishers
90 Fifth Avenue
New York, New York 10011
Copyright © 1988 by Frederick T. Zugibe
All rights reserved. No part of this book
may be reproduced, in any form, without written
permission from the publisher, unless by a reviewer
who wishes to quote brief passages.

Library of Congress Cataloging-in-Publication Data

Zugibe, Frederick T.
The cross and the shroud.   9-88

    Bibliography: p.
    Includes index.
    1. Jesus Christ—Crucifixion.   2. Holy Shroud.
3. Forensic pathology.   4. Crucifixion—Physiological
aspects.   I. Title.   [DNLM: 1. Jesus Christ.   2. Death.
Forensic Medicine.   W 800 Z94c]
BT450.283. 1988   232.9'63   87-15688
ISBN 0-913729-75-2
ISBN 0-913729-46-9 (pbk.)

Contents

Illustrations

Preface

Read not to contradict and confute, nor
to believe and take for granted . . . .
but to weigh and consider.

FRANCIS BACON, *Essays: of Studies*

   This book represents the culmination of thirty-eight years of research into the medical aspects of crucifixion. My original interest in the Shroud of Turin was primarily to obtain information regarding mechanisms and cause of death in crucifixion. In this regard, authenticity of the Shroud was very important because, if the Shroud was determined to be an authentic shroud of a crucified being near the time of Jesus, the information would be of inestimable value in determining the type of suffering and the mechanisms and cause of death in crucifixion. This investigation was by far the most challenging and intriguing experience that I have ever encountered either as a full-time forensic pathologist-medical examiner or as a medical research scientist. During my career as a medical examiner, I have encountered many puzzling and bizarre homicides, complicated auto accident cases, and intricate body identifications; yet none compared to the intricacies that confronted me during my probe into the demise of Jesus. This experience constituted a formidable challenge to my entire scientific and medical background in forensic pathology, medicine, anatomy, biochemistry, inorganic and organic chemistry, electron microscopy, biophysics, physiology, and botany.
   Since the 1978 Exposition of the Shroud in Turin, Italy, and

subsequent scientific studies of the Shroud, the field of Shroud studies has expanded in breathtaking fashion, making it extremely difficult for the dilettante or untrained novice to separate the chaff from the wheat. Multitudes of articles have been published by sincere individuals whose intentions were good, but who did not possess the necessary education, training, and experience in forensic pathology to evaluate and interpret the materials and to render valid conclusions, or who, influenced by their religious fervor, reached erroneous and untenable suppositions and conclusions, *argumentum ad hominem.* I meet this well-intentioned but weakly supported presentation frequently in court cases when I testify as an expert witness regarding scientific or medical facts. The trial attorneys frequently impress the jury with their apparently vast knowledge of the scientific or medical facts and scientific literature they had memorized a few days before trial. The unfortunate part is that they frequently do not know the fine points that are a sine qua non for proper understanding of the problem.

This is essentially a complete update of my book, *The Cross and the Shroud, A Medical Examiner Investigates the Crucifixion* (Angelus Books). The various sections have been either completely rewritten, expanded or eliminated in light of more recent studies, or corrections have been made where problems have been resolved. The latest findings, from the 1978 Exposition to the present, are incorporated within the various sections, and new photographs and illustrations have been added. In the following chapters, I have attempted to investigate the sufferings and death of Jesus, the images on the Turin Shroud, and the results of scientific and other research studies in the same objective and questioning manner I used to investigate scores of forensic cases as part of my duties as forensic pathologist and chief medical examiner. Moreover, meticulous experiments were conducted in an endeavor to resolve critical areas of controversies that have been propagated *idées fixes* such as the asphyxiation theory, the sites of transfixion to the cross, blood flow concepts, etc. Moreover, I have attempted to show the errors in major concepts currently being quoted ad infinitum such as the asphyxiation hypothesis, Destot's space concept, the double flow of blood on the wrist hypothesis, the drawing in of the thumb hypothesis, the man of the Shroud was not washed concept, the nail through the wrist theory, and certain image theories as the hyperthermia-calcium carbonate concept, the precipitation of silver concept, iron oxide concept, and others.

Many scientific concepts are very complex. In this regard, I have made every effort to present the subject matter in a form that would be understandable to the reader with no training in the medical or scientific fields and at the same time be acceptable to the probing mind of the trained scientist.

The
CROSS
and the
SHROUD

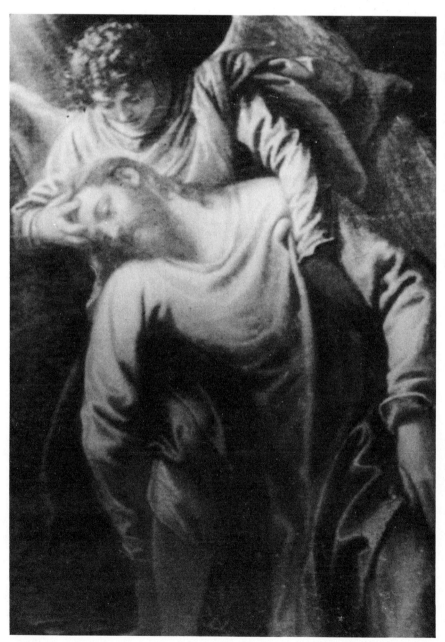

Figure 1-1
Agony in the Garden.
Renaissance painting, unknown artist.

1

The Agony in the Garden of Olives

On the night of the Pasch, along the road from Jerusalem to Bethany, somewhere beyond the Kidron Valley on the western slope of the Mount of Olives, referred to as Gethsemane, a spectacle of monumental significance was taking place. With an unsteady gait, Jesus of Nazareth appeared, deeply saddened, and in a trembling voice addressed his three favorite Apostles: Peter, James, and John. "My soul is very sorrowful, even unto death, remain here and watch" (Mark 14:34). This was unlike the Jesus they had witnessed during his Transfiguration a short time ago. After a period of utter exhaustion and repeated praying, he looked up to heaven and said, "'Father, if thou art willing, remove this cup from me: nevertheless, not my will but yours be done.' And there appeared to him an angel from heaven, strengthening him, and being in agony, he prayed more earnestly and his sweat became like great drops of blood falling down upon the ground." (Luke 22:42–44). St. Luke, the author of this passage, was a physician and a Greek native of Antioch, who wrote in the Districts of Achaia and Boeotia. He was well educated, knew Aramaic, and was conversant with Greco-Roman and Jewish culture. He had completed his medical studies at Tarsus and was a close companion to St. Paul. He drew his information primarily from eyewitnesses and documents and wrote his Gospel about A.D. 61, although some sources relate it as far as A.D. 63. Luke was an accurate historian whose style was elegant, with a smooth flow of language and a prodigious vocabulary. It appears strange that none

1

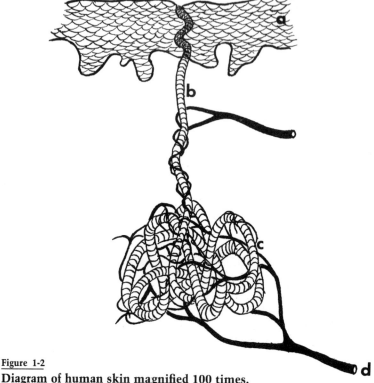

Figure 1-2

Diagram of human skin magnified 100 times.
(a) *Epidermis (top layer of skin).*
(b) *duct (tubule) of the sweat gland.*
(c) *coiled sweat gland (eccrine).*
(d) *blood supply of sweat gland.*

of the other Gospels contain information on either the sweating of blood or the comforting angel. It must be realized, however, that Luke was a physician and probably was more sensitive to any bits of medical or scientific facts reported by the three Apostles who accompanied Christ in the Garden of Gethsemane and would have carefully queried his sources of information for accuracy. Unfortunately, many of the early Christians deliberately left out material regarding these two points because of an unfounded fear of the early enemies of Christianity, such as Celsus and Porphyry, who attacked the credibility of the Gospels. Later, when these fears were put to rest, numerous Codices of the early writers reinstated them in a manner that leaves not a shadow of a doubt as to the authenticity of this passage.

HEMATIDROSIS

(Sudorcruentus, Sudor Sanguineus, hemorrhagia percutem, Hematidrose, Suerdesany)

St. Luke's account of the Agony in the Garden has plagued rationalists and theologians for centuries as to whether this was merely a figurative expression or whether it was possible for a human to sweat blood.

In regard to the first query, there is no reason to believe that Luke meant his words figuratively because there is no logical meaning to the expression. For example, if one said, "like water dripping from a leaky faucet" or "like raindrops," then there would be a figurative meaning. A figurative interpretation truly is not possible, according to the rules of language, because we cannot use it in a new sense apparently for the purpose of controversy.

The last query is the proper one because there is a rare medical disorder called hematidrosis, which is defined in *Stedman's Medical Dictionary* as an excretion of blood or blood pigments in the sweat. Early references to this physiological phenomenon include the observation by Aristotle, "some sweat with a bloody sweat" (*Hist. Animal* III, 19). Hematidrosis was also referred to in Hobart's *Medical Language of St. Luke* (1882). Dr. Ryland Whittaker, in his article "The Physical Cause of the Death of Our Lord," and LeBec, in his "The Death of the Cross," both found several instances on record of hematidrosis. LeBec indicated that in many of the cases red blood corpuscles were clearly revealed under the microscope.

The reported cases of hematidrosis appeared to be associated with a severe anxiety reaction with fear implicated as the inciting factor. Cases of hematidrosis have been reported in the French literature by Broeg in 1907 and by Darier in 1930; in the British literature in 1918 by Scott, in the German literature by Riecke in 1923, and in the Russian literature by Lavsky in 1932 and by Gadzhiev and Listengarten in 1962. Scott relates a case of an intelligent young girl of eleven who was sheltered by her parents because she was very nervous about air raids. She had frequent bouts of hematidrosis that began a week after a very severe shock when she became frightened by a gas explosion that had occurred in the next house while she was in bed. Gadzhiev and Listengarten studied a case of hematidrosis in a young woman who began sweating blood at nineteen years of age. This frequently occurred when the patient was nervous, excited, worried and scared. Lav-sky's case was also associated with psychological changes. In all the cases, red blood corpuscles were observed under the microscope. No blood or other physical abnormalities were found following examination to account for the phenomenon, and the disorder did not appear to be amenable to treatment.

ANATOMICAL CONSIDERATIONS

To understand the mechanism of hematidrosis, it is necessary to learn some basic facts regarding the sweat glands. First, there are essentially two types of sweat glands, exocrine glands and apocrine glands. The former are the primary sweat glands, which are dis-tributed all over the surface of the body and, according to various studies, account for over two million glands. They are smaller in size than the apocrine sweat glands and consist of tubular, coiled glands situated well beneath the skin as indicated in Figure 1-2. These glands are completely coiled and entwined by numerous blood vessels, as indicated in Figures 1-3 and 1-4. The tubules are ducts that carry the sweat to the outside surface of the skin. The apocrine sweat glands are large sweat glands that do not occur over the whole body, but are restricted to the axillary (underarm) region, an area below the umbilicus, the breast region, the midline of the abdomen, the genital region, the ear canal, and the opening of the nose. These latter glands apparently are derived from hair follicle cells. Only on very rare occasions have some of these glands occurred on the face.

The fact of sweating is governed by the autonomic nervous system, which consists of the sympathetic (SD) and parasym-pathetic divisions (PD). These control various bodily functions, such as heart rate, movements of the gastrointestinal tract, caliber of blood vessels, sweating, contraction or relaxation of muscles of the urinary bladder, gallbladder, and bronchi, regulation of the pupils of the eye, and accommodation. For practical purposes, these two divisions may be regarded as being antagonistic to one another, i.e. they counteract the effect of each other. For example, the SD increases the heart rate during excitement, and the PD slows it down. The SD relaxes or dilates the pupil to let in more light during dusk, and the PD constricts (narrows) the pupil in the direct sunlight to reduce the amount of light entering the eyes. The SD relaxes the eye for far vision, and the PD contracts the eye for

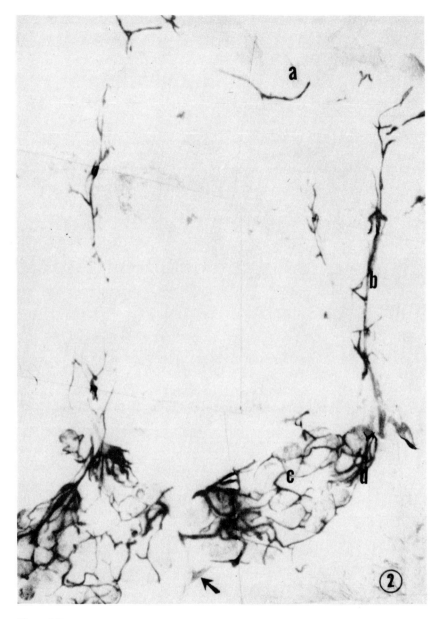

Figure 1-3

Photo of human skin under a microscope magnified sixty times.
(a) epidermis (top layer of skin).
(b) duct (tubule) of the sweat gland.
(c) coiled sweat gland (eccrine).
(d) blood supply of sweat gland.
(Courtesy of W. Montagna, Oregon Regional Primate Research Center, Beaverton, Oregon.)

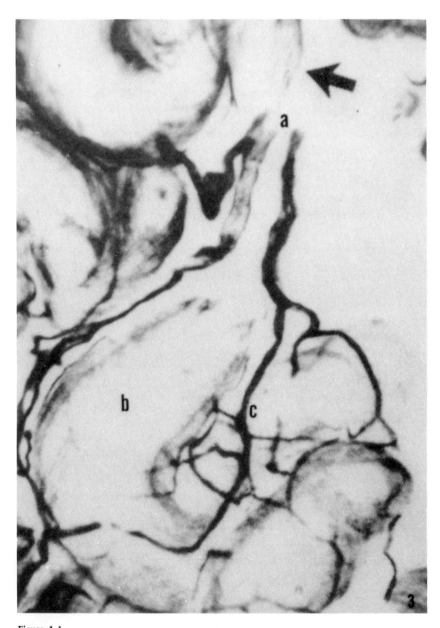

Figure 1-4

Photo of human skin taken under a microscope magnified 100 times.

(a) duct (tubule) of the sweat gland.

(b) area within the sweat gland.

(c) blood vessels surroundng the sweat gland.

Note the proximity of the blood vessels to the inside of the sweat glands.

(Permission of W. Montagna, Oregon Regional Primate Research Center, Beaverton, Oregon.)

near vision. Now, how does this relate to the initiation of the phenomenon of hematidrosis? First, a severely stressful situation from either emotional or physical causes initiates the defense-alarm reaction or the famous "fight or flight reaction," which causes activation of sympathetic activity where adrenalin is primarily produced and the heart rate is accelerated, the blood vessels constrict, blood is diverted away from the skin, the blood vessels and skeletal muscle become dilated to increase vision, blood sugar increases, and oxygen consumption increases. The initiating factor in the Garden of Gethsemane was the turbulent water of sadness, extreme fear, and anxious trepidation, which were taxing his spirit to the extreme limits of his humanity. "My soul is exceedingly sorrowful unto death." His mission was clear, and he was able to envision the entire gamut of suffering: "Father, if thou art willing, remove this cup from me: nevertheless not my will, but thine, be done" (Luke 22:42). Also, the fact that Christ "fell on the ground, and prayed . . ." (Mark 14:35) was indicative of his weakness because it was unusual for a Jew to kneel during prayer. This prelude satisfies all of the medical criteria of extreme fear to invoke this sympathetic autonomic response. Christ prayed over and over and over again. This severe response was followed by a counter-response initiated by the parasympathetic nervous system. Probably when "there appeared an angel unto him from heaven (Figure 1-1) strengthening him" (Luke 22:43), he had accepted his fate. The heart rate slowed, there was marked sweating over the entire body, his muscles relaxed, and blood rushed back into the delicate capillaries that were in close apposition to the sweat gland lumina (Figures 1-2 and 1-3), causing the vessels to rupture into the sweat gland, thence mixing with the sweat and extruding to the surface of the skin through the coiled tubules. The increased production of sweat forced the blood, mixed with sweat, through the tubules (ducts) to the outside surface of the skin, where they would emerge from the ducts as drops falling to the ground. I do not, however, believe that clotting occurred on contact with the air, because blood does not usually clot that rapidly unless there was some severe alteration in the clotting mechanism. Since hematidrosis is a rare phenomenon, it may have appeared as clots of blood to the observer. Another possibility is that something may have been lost in translation regarding the word "clot" because the word "drop" would be more logical. I do not, however, believe that this is an important point.

CHROMHIDROSIS

A new school of thought that has gained impetus in recent years attributes the sweating of blood to a condition called chromhidrosis, which is characterized by the secretion of a colored sweat. This theory is untenable but is worthy of discussion primarily to dispel it. The proponents of this hypothesis include Shelley and Hurley, who reviewed the literature, cited cases of chromhidrosis, and suggested a relationship to localized hematidrosis to explain the bleeding phenomenon manifested by stigmatics. Dr. Rothman, in his book, the *Physiology and Biochemistry of the Skin,* agreed that this was a significant point, and he appeared to suggest that the bleeding palms of Theresa of Konnersreuth, the Austrian stigmatic, may be explained on the basis of colored sweat. He admits that it was improbable in the case of Theresa of Konnersreuth, because the occurrence of apocrine glands in the palms would be unlikely for phylogenetic reasons and, moreover, Theresa never secreted a bloody sweat of the palms. She displayed hemorrhagic wounds of the back and front of the hands. Professor Ewald, a professor of psychiatry at the University of Erlangen, who observed one of her episodes, reported a scab-covered, tender, hemorrhagic lesion of the back of the hands and feet, with smaller lesions on corresponding spots of the palm and soles, as well as over the heart next to the sternum. This certainly is not related to a sweating phenomenon. Shelley and Hurley referred to the hippopotamus, which is famed for "sweating blood" but actually excretes a red, sticky, apocrine sweaty substance when angered or otherwise excited. I contacted Professor C. P. Luck of the Department of Physiology of the Makere University College Medical School in Kampala, Uganda, whom I believe to be one of the most knowledgeable scientists in the world regarding the physiology of the sweat glands of the hippopotamus. He said it usually sweats a red substance, but not always, and this is certainly not restricted to episodes of anger, as was indicated by Shelley and Hurley. He further indicated that hippos do not usually sweat during or following anger, and it is an individual matter. Because this phenomenon does exist in the hippo, I scanned the entire medical literature but was unable to find a single case of a person with chromhidrosis who had ever secreted a red secretion anywhere on the body, particularly the face. Even if one or two people were found, it would certainly be difficult to attribute this phenomenon to Christ. If one would merely use logical reasoning, this theory as related to Christ can easily be dispelled, because there was absolutely no mention made of Christ sweating blood by any of the throngs of people who observed Christ's crucifixion when he was sweating rivers of sweat. Certainly, if Christ had chromhidrosis, it would have been grossly apparent to everyone.

THE IMPORTANCE OF THE AGONY IN THE GARDEN

In order to fully realize the consequences of Jesus' agony in the Garden of Gethsemane, it is necessary to understand the effects of anxiety on the body.

Anxiety is defined by Adams and Hope as a medical phenomenon that "designates a state characterized by a subjective feeling of fear and uneasy anticipation (apprehension) usually with a definite topical content and associated with the physiological accompaniments of fear, i.e.; breathlessness, choking sensation, palpitation, restlessness, increased muscular tension, tightness in the chest, giddiness, trembling, sweating, flushing, and broken sleep."

Much has been written on the physiological and psychological bases of anxiety states, but many hold to the theory that anxiety is based on fear as an inherited instinctual pattern, is a response to a situation of danger, and is internally based somewhere in the unconscious.

Anxiety states are of two major varieties: the acute attack, which has a duration of a few minutes to hours, and the chronic type, which may last from hours to years. The acute anxiety attacks provoke an intense fear of dying accompanied by loss of reason, palpitations, sweating, tremulousness, choking sensation, pallor, and shortness of breath. I have seen many individuals in such a state who were brought to the hospital by ambulance under the mistaken assumption that they were the victims of heart attack.

Anxiety and depression cause terribly uncomfortable feelings that incessantly gnaw at individuals, frequently disabling or incapacitating them or throwing them into a state of panic. These acute attacks are called anxiety attacks. Fatigue is a frequent consequence of the increased effort of attempting to cope with the distressing fear. Some of the symptoms include irritability, apprehension, insomnia, agitation, pallor, changes in heart rate, inner tremulousness, palpitations, inability to concentrate, and loss of appetite. The individual may become startled at the slightest unexpected stimulus, and a hopeless state frequently pervades the entire being of the individual, immobilizing him or causing episodes of uncontrollable crying. People who are under such mental anguish develop lowered spirits, have feelings of dejection, feel melancholy, become withdrawn, and depict undue sadness, lassitude, despair, discouragement, and lack of ambition. We frequently hear people who are undergoing a severe emotional crisis, because of severe illness or death of a loved one, relate that they would rather have physical pain than the unrelenting, gnawing mental anxiety that they are suffering. Some who are unable to cope with their problems become preoccupied with suicide, and if this is not recognized and treated early, the result may be disastrous.

A case in point involves a forty-year-old man with a cancer phobia who was awaiting the results of laboratory tests because he was convinced that he had cancer. On Sunday morning, he noted a small "lump" under his arm and called his doctor in a state of panic. The doctor examined him and assured him that it probably was not cancer. The man stopped eating and hyperventilated repeatedly, resulting in lightheadedness and tingling of his fingers, which he interpreted as spread of the imaginary cancer. He would lie on the sofa for six to eight hours at a time and then pace the floor. His nights were sleepless, and during the next few days he became severely fatigued with palpitations. When he went back to the doctor who biopsied the lesion, he was informed that the lump appeared totally benign and he would have the final results in a few days. The next two days were "Hell on Earth" with pacing of the floor, severe sweating episodes, and lying in an almost comatose state. His brother came home the day after the biopsy to find that the man had hanged himself. The irony was that the mass was diagnosed as a benign cyst.

It is of profound importance to realize that the full impact of the Agony in the Garden is not generally recognized among Christians. Its significance derives from the realization that Christ not only displayed severe physical suffering during the Way of the Cross, but that he also previously suffered severe mental anguish that drains or attenuates the physical strength of an individual to the point of total exhaustion.

The overall effects of this extreme mental suffering that Jesus had undergone with the consequent hematidrosis and lack of sleep would have been significant in causing his final demise. Therefore, an understanding of the suffering of Christ in the Garden of

Gethsemane is paramount to fully appreciate why Pilate was surprised that Christ died as early as he did. At the time of his condemnation, he had no knowledge of Christ's Agony in the Garden.

> Reproach hath broken my heart; and I am full of heaviness: and I looked *for some* to take pity, but *there was* none; and for comforters, but I found none.
>
> Psalms 69:20

2

The Scourging

THE TRIAL OF JESUS

It was about 2 A.M. when Jesus
was bound and led away from the Garden of Gethsemane by a
detachment of temple attendants and Roman soldiers across the
Kidron Valley to the home of Caiaphas, the high priest, where he
was to appear before the Sanhedrin early in the morning. Following
a preliminary interrogation by Annas, father-in-law of Caiaphas,
Jesus was taken to a holding area where "the men who were holding
Jesus mocked him and beat him. 'Prophesy: Who is it that struck
you?' And they spoke other words against him" (Luke 22:63–65). A
few hours later, as the dawn was breaking, the fatigued and humili-
ated Jesus was brought before the Sanhedrin, the highest religious
body of the land, presided over by Caiaphas. This body was composed of the high priests, the leaders of the people, and the
Pharisees and scribes. This hearing failed to provide the normal
prerequisites for a conviction according to Jewish law, which man-
dates that the testimony of at least two witnesses is necessary for a
condemnation of death and not merely the testimony of the accused (Deut. 17:6, 19:15; Num. 3:30). Caiaphas asked Jesus, "Are
you the Christ, the son of the Blessed?" And Jesus said, "I am, and
you will see the son of man sitting at the right hand of power and
coming with the clouds of Heaven" (Mark 14:62). This was all they

12

had to hear; the Sanhedrin quickly condemned him to death without regard to witnesses because they considered his divine claim of being the Messiah as blasphemy. The procurator of Judea, however, was the only person empowered to order the death sentence, and they knew that their only hope for his approval would be on a political basis and not on the religious charge. "Then led they Jesus from Caiaphas unto the hall of judgment" (John 18:28) to appear before Pilate. The praetorium (hall of judgment) was the place where the praetor discharged his duties in the *lithostrotos* or "pavement" at the Roman fortress of *Antonia* located on the "highest of hills" (Josephus, *Jewish War*). This fortress was composed of four towers, which enclosed a large courtyard. The chief priests and scribes brought Jesus before the procurator of Judea, Pontius Pilate, the *Jusgladii*, "And they began to accuse him, saying, 'We found this *fellow* perverting the nation and forbidding to give tribute to Caesar, saying that he himself is Christ a King'" (Luke 23:2). "He stirreth up the people, teaching throughout all Jewry, beginning from Galilee to this place" (Luke 23:5). Jesus was then led inside, and Pilate reentered the praetorium and took his place on the *curule* chair in the center of the high, arched tribunal. After quizzing Jesus, he indicated to these people that he could find no crime Jesus had committed and certainly no *lese majeste* against Rome. Pilate even tried to get rid of the whole affair by sending him to Herod after he found that Jesus was a Galilean and under Herod's jurisdiction, but Herod merely arrayed him in gorgeous apparel and sent him back to Pilate. At this time, Pilate still insisted that Christ was not guilty of the charges, and Pilate had no intentions of killing him because, he related, "Behold, nothing deserving death has been done by him. I will, therefore, chastise him and release him" (Luke 13:15–16). He then ordered the scourging with the intention of appeasing the chief priests and the rulers of the Jewish people because he assumed that once they beheld Jesus in such a wretched state, *ecce homo*, it would quell their punitive desires. "Then Pilate therefore took Jesus, and scourged *him*" (John 19:1).

But what actually is the act of scourging? How is it executed, and what effects would it have on the victim? Many people conceive of scourging as a mere beating with a whip. In a sense, this is true. But it is, however, like comparing an electric shock to a lightning bolt.

WHAT IS SCOURGING?

Scourging or *flagellatio* was a form of brutal, inhumane punishment generally effected by Roman soldiers using the dreaded and most feared instrument of the time, called a flagrum or, in the words of Horatio, "the horrible flagellum." This was made in various forms, the most common being a leather whip containing several leather tails or thongs with small weights of metal or bone at the end of each tail (Figure 2-1).

In rare cases, the weights were pointed and referred to as *scorpiones*. Another type of flagrum was a whiplike structure containing three chains. Some contained small weights or buttonlike

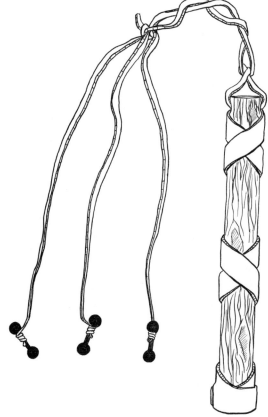

Figure 2-1
The Roman flagrum.
Composed of leather tails containing small weights of metal or bone. The dumbbell shape of the weights corresponds to the configurations made on the Turin Shroud. (See Figure 2-3.)

objects. Most of the evidence indicates that the multitail flagrum with rounded bits of metal or bone was used prior to crucifixion. Although the number of lashes in some instances was determined by the whims of the executioner, the victim was usually given only a few lashes. They did not want him to succumb too quickly for that would interfere with the act of crucifixion. The number of lashes also depended on who the individual was. Traitors and political prisoners were crucified for long periods of time so that the crowds could behold the errors of these persons' ways. Scourging was sometimes used as a form of capital punishment, where the victim was beaten to death, and also as a means of extracting information from spies, political prisoners, and those trying to overcome the government. Usually, the greater the crime, the more cruel the punishment with the flagrum, except in the case of crucifixion, where, as was previously related, it was not intended for the individual to die too quickly on the cross. In some instances, the victim was scourged on the way to crucifixion. Scourging is not to be confused with another type of punishment that the Romans utilized, called *verberatio,* purported to have a much lesser effect, where rods were used instead of the flagrum. An instance of this type was explicitly related in Verven 554, where Servillius, a Roman citizen, was subjected to a beating by several men with rods. The beating was very severe, whereupon he collapsed, but the beating was continued until he purportedly gave his word. He died a short while later.

THE ACT OF SCOURGING

The victim was usually stripped naked and shackled by the wrists to a low column, causing him to assume a bent position to make the executioner's task easier. One or more Roman soldiers were delegated the task of initiating the flogging. The soldier would stand holding the flagrum by the side of the prisoner and, upon command, would draw the leather instrument toward his back, rotate his wrist, and lash it in an arclike fashion across the naked back. The weight of the metal or bone objects frequently carried them to the front of the body (Figure 2-2). In addition, the shoulders, arms, and legs down to and including the calves were lashed. The bits of metal dug deep into the flesh, ripping small blood vessels, nerves, muscle, and skin. This maneuver was repeated over and over again, with the soldier changing position to the opposite side periodically until the allotted number of lashes were given. Large black and blue and reddish-purple welts and swellings appeared all over the front and back of the victim's body, primarily around the puncture marks made by the bits of metal. The victim writhed and twisted in agony, falling to his knees, only to be jerked back on his feet time and time again until he could no longer stand up. Bouts of vomiting, tremors, seizures, and fainting fits occurred at varying intervals and sometimes appeared concomitantly during these maneuvers. There were agonizing shrieks by the victim at the conclusion of each lash, usually with begging and pleading for mercy. The victim was reduced to an exhausted, mangled mass of flesh with a craving for water. He was in a state of traumatic shock.

THE MOSAIC LAW

It is of interest to note that it was against Mosaic Law to exceed forty lashes, and thirty-nine were usually given so that the

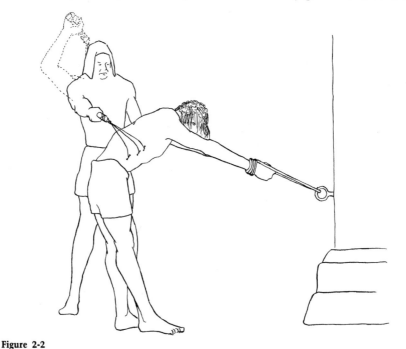

Figure 2-2
The act of scourging.
The victim was shackled to a low column, and the Roman soldier would provide the number of lashes across the naked back of the victim as ordered.

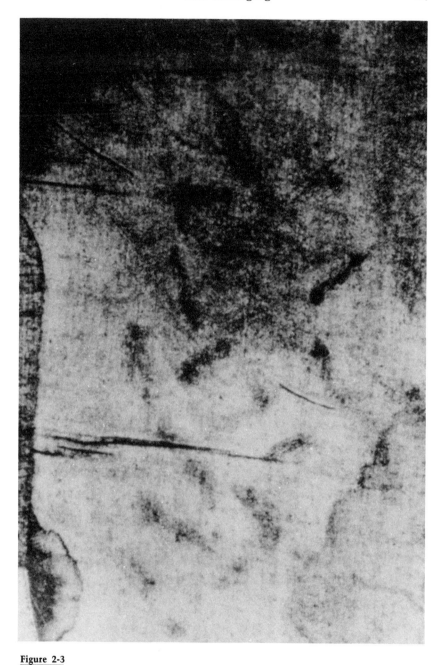

Figure 2-3
Shroud of Turin, back area.
This is a blow up of the scourge marks. The marks are relatively well defined and some show a dumbbell shape corresponding to the weights of the flagrum. (See Figure 2-1.)

law was not exceeded. This is stated in Deuteronomy 25:3: where it states that "Forty stripes may be given him, but not more; lest, if one should go on to beat him with more stripes than these, your brother be degraded in your sight." Also, in 2 Corinthians 11:24, "five times I have received at the hands of the Jews the forty lashes less one." For Christ it was, however, a different situation, because the Roman soldiers would decide how many lashes to inflict. This would depend on various factors, such as the prisoner's endurance, the nature of his crime, their mood, the wishes of the crowd, and, of course, in the capital form of punishment, they would lash the individual until he died.

In the case of Christ, Pilate's order to have him scourged was based on his desire to appease the crowd lest they denounce him to the emperor or even start a revolt against him. This was a solely political move on the part of Pilate, because both he and Herod found no guilt, and therefore how could he even subject Jesus to the most feared of all punishments—the Roman *flagellatio?* This obviously did not appease anyone, because even when Pilate gave the Jewish officials the option of releasing a murderer and thief by the name of Barabbas, he was sure that they would not want a killer in their midst and would certainly take Jesus; but they cried out that they wanted to release Barabbas and they wanted Christ crucified. Therefore, Pilate had no other choice but to pronounce sentence, which was irrevocable. *Ibis ad crucem* (Thou shalt go to the cross).

EVIDENCE FROM THE TURIN SHROUD

An analysis of the Shroud of Turin very strikingly reveals dumbbell-shaped markings all over the front and back of the trunk and legs, essentially sparing the head, neck, and distal aspects of the extremities consistent with the use of bits of metal or bone on the end of a flagrum. The number of scourge impressions totals from 100 to 120 (Figure 2-3). Some scientists, who have studied the Shroud in detail, indicate that the various markings on the Shroud are directed downward and inward toward the center of the body, suggesting either that two individuals executed the scourging or that one individual changed his position from one side to the other.

3

The Crown of Thorns

THE KING OF THE JEWS

The pitiable looking, inhumanely beaten Jesus, whose body was severely distorted and racked with pain from the terrifying scourging, his vision blurred, barely able to stand, was led into the praetorium by the soldiers, where "they clothed him in a purple cloak and plaiting a crown of thorns, they put it on him and they began to salute him, 'Hail King of the Jews' and they struck his head with a reed and spat upon him" (Mark 15:17–19).

After all, had he not claimed to be King of the Jews? This was all the soldiers needed. They called in all of their cohorts, where they created a hilarious parody or burlesque of his kingship. This ludicrous imitation included a purple cloak, the imperial purple symbolizing royalty or high esteem in which they held him. Kings and victorious leaders wore such vestments following major victories. In addition, they plaited a crown of thorns in the form of a cap and placed it on his head to continue the mock coronation. The burlesque continued by placing a reed in his hand as a scepter. The soldiers filed past Christ, kneeling before him, spitting on him, and striking him with the reed against the crown of thorns, the nose, and the face, as they paid false homage to him (an imitation of Ave Caesar Imperator). His face was bruised and his nose broken. What fun they were having and how they attempted to ridicule him for their own enjoyment!

The significance of the mock coronation is that the crowning of thorns was in actuality a major source of suffering not generally appreciated by Christians. Unfortunately, the emphasis regarding the crowning of thorns has always been placed on the gross humiliation that Christ was subjected to rather than on the pain he suffered. The effect of this type of pain was probably not understood by Pilate because parodies of this type were not a usual prelude to crucifixion, and none have ever been related in the vast literature on crucifixion.

WHAT TYPE OF SUFFERING WOULD BE INFLICTED
BY THE CROWN OF THORNS?

Before we can answer this question, it is necessary to understand something about the nature of the plant utilized to plait the crown, the anatomy of the head region, and an explanation of the medical entities that are closely related.

THE ORIGIN OF THE CROWN OF THORNS

The plant used in plaiting the crown of thorns has been the subject of much debate. But the most renowned botanical experts on the flora of the Holy Land have narrowed down the prospects to either the Syrian Christ thorn (*Ziziphus spina christi* L. Wild.), also known as *Rhamnus spina christi* (L.) and *Rhamnus nabeca Forsk* (Figure 3-1, 3-2), or Christ's thorn *Paliuris spina christi* (Mill.), also known as *Paliuris aculeatus* (Lam.) or *Rhamnus paliuris* (L. Wild.) and *Ziziphus paliuris* (L.) (Figure 3-2). Both of these plants are members of the Buckthorn family (*Rhamnaceae*) and closely resemble each other. The Syrian Christ thorn is also known as the *dom*, *sidr*, or *nulok*, and according the Moldenke, "grows abundantly on the plains from Syria and Lebanon through Palestine to Arabia, Petraea, and Sinai." Dr. Michael Evenari, professor at the Hebrew University of Jerusalem, indicated to me in his correspondence that Christ's thorn is a northern Mediterranean species found on the southern border of Israel and to some extent in Samaria, but is not found today in Jerusalem or its surroundings. He related that it is improbable that it grew in Jerusalem during Christ's time but admits that no one can be certain. On the other hand, he was of

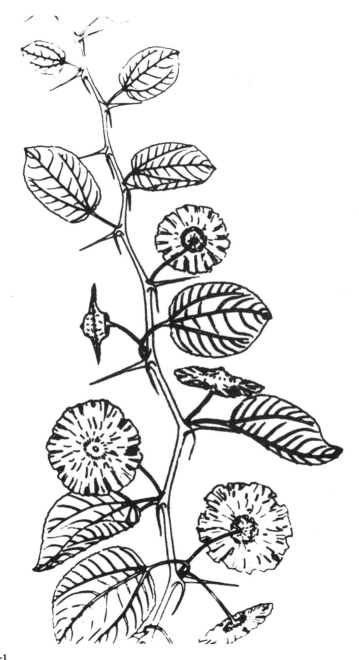

Figure 3-1
Syrian Christ Thorn (Ziziphus spina Christi L. Wild).
A pair of stout, unequal, curved *spines with sharp points are present at the base of each leaf.*

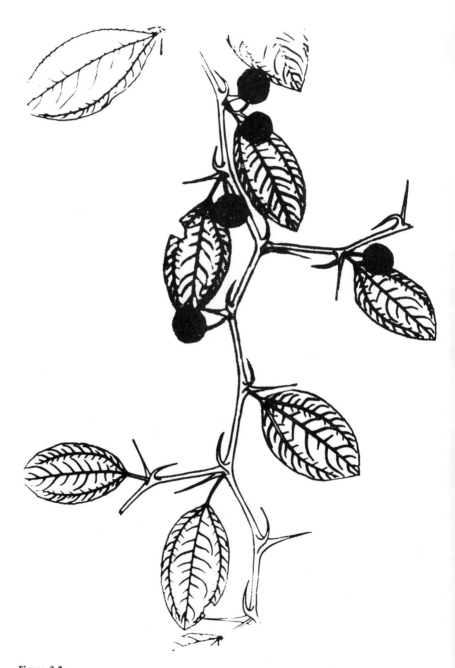

Figure 3-2
Christ's Thorn (Paliurus spina Christi Mill.).
A pair of unequal, very stiff, sharp, stipular spines are present, with one of each curved and shorter than the other.

the opinion that the Syrian Christ thorn was a more likely candidate and was more common than the Christ's thorn. The botanist G. Post agrees with Dr. Evenari, does not record Christ's thorn in Jerusalem, and indicates that it does not grow in Judea. He does record it in other areas about the Holy Land including Nazareth, Galilee, Jaffa, and Beirut. The great Linnaeus gave his opinion that the Syrian Christ thorn was the plant out of which the crown of thorns was made. Authors such as Tristram and Warburger, as quoted by Hegi, have taken the opposite view and are of the opinion that it was common about Jerusalem. Zohary disagrees with Hegi, maintaining that Christ's thorn is not a Mediterranean plant. The pliability and ease of plaiting a crown is perhaps the reason why many of the authors were partial to Christ's thorn, but, because both plants are very similar morphologically, it makes little difference which of the two was used.

Both the Syrian Christ thorn and the Christ's thorn are characterized by closely spaced, sharp thorns as described above and have been plaited inherently, adding a greater surface area of thorns per unit of skin contact. The Syrian Christ thorn is a shrub that grows from nine to fifteen feet tall and contains smooth white branches with a pair of stout, unequal, recurved spines at the base of each leaf. The leaves appear leathery and are ovate to elliptical and contain small greenish-colored flowers in small clusters. The Christ's thorn is a shrub that grows between three and nine feet tall, contains a pair of unequal, very stiff, sharp, stipular spines with one of each pair of the spines being curved and shorter than the other one. The leaves are also leathery and from oval to round in shape.

OTHER IMPLICATED PLANTS

It is important to note that the popular greenhouse plant that widely adorns the homes of Christians, known commonly as the crown of thorns (*Euphorea splendens* or *milii*), is native to Madagascar and did not grow in the Holy Land during the time of Christ. This is a sprawling, branching, vinelike plant with angular stems and brilliant scarlet-colored flower bracts just below the true flowers. This flower is a member of the *Euphorabaceae*. It has absolutely nothing to do with the plants of the Bible. *Zizyphus officinarum* (Medic.), known as the jujube, a prodigious fruit-bearing plant, had been implicated but it has been precluded, because, although it is cultivated in the region, it was brought from China or India and it is not believed native to Palestine and Syria. Other plants that have been implicated include *Koeberlinia spinosa*, *Canotia holacantha* (mojave thorn), *Holocantha emoryi*, and *Dalea spinosa*. None of these plants had anything to do with the biblical plants used to make the crown of thorns. Unfortunately, many devout Christians tenaciously believe one plant or another to be implicated and are not swayed by reasoning. An interesting story in this regard is told by the renowned botanist F. Schwerin, who visited the Garden of Gethsemane in the early part of this century. A monk in charge pointed to a shrub growing there, which was the plant called *Gleditsia tricanthos* L. (honey locust, sweet locust, thorny locust), and informed Schwerin that it was the plant from which the crown of thorns was originally made. Even though Schwerin told the monk that the plant was an American species unknown at the time of Christ, the monk replied that two female pilgrims originally brought it in a flowerpot and asserted that he was more inclined to believe the devout women than a mere botanist.

ANATOMICAL CONSIDERATIONS OF THE HEAD REGION

The head region is extremely vascular, that is, it contains myriads of blood vessels so that even small wounds cause marked bleeding episodes. The nerve supply for pain perception is distributed by branches of two major nerves: the trigeminal nerve, which essentially supplies the front half of the head, and the greater occipital branch, which supplies the back half of the head (Figure 3-3). Only a schematic representation of the nerve distribution is shown because the fine nervous branches divide almost infinitesimally throughout the skin. To appreciate this distribution, take a pin and attempt to find a spot on your scalp that is pain-free. You will soon realize that it is an almost impossible task.

Stimulation of any of the branches of these nerves causes pain. For example, if any of the very tiny branches of the trigeminal nerve that supply the teeth are irritated, a toothache is initiated, and everyone knows the pain associated with a toothache. It is certainly difficult to believe that irritation of such a tiny nerve twig could cause so much pain. Another major clinical entity associated with irritation of the trigeminal nerve is a condition of unknown cause called *tic douloureux* or major trigeminal neuralgia, first described by Fothergill in 1776, which causes paroxysmal bouts of

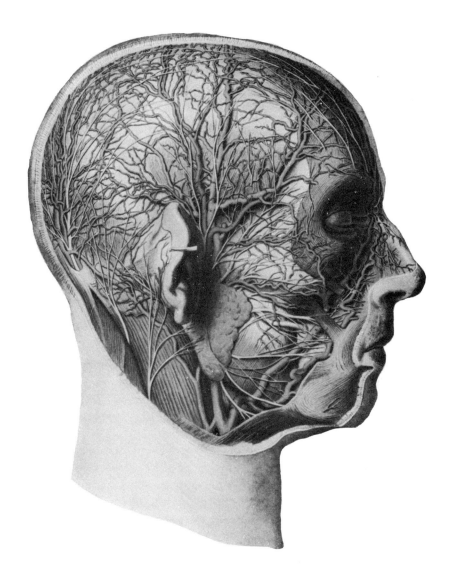

Figure 3-3
Diagram of the head region.
*Shows nerve distribution (light colored branches) and blood vessels (dark
branches).*
(Permission of Urban and Schwartzenberg, Munich, West Germany, from Atlas of
Descriptive Anatomy *by Sobotta, Fig. 56.)*

stabbing, lancinating, explosive paroxysmal pains of the right or left half of the face lasting from seconds to minutes with intermittent refractory periods. Although it is characteristic for patients to be free of pain between paroxysms, instances of pain may at times occur in such rapid succession that a sustained background ache develops. Trigger zones or pain-provoking areas are usually present on a lip or side of the nose and can be activated by tactile stimulation. If such an area is touched or struck, a paroxysm of severe pain occurs that immobilizes the individual. Patients describe their pains as "knifelike stabs," "electric shocks," or "jabs with a red hot poker." During the attack, tics or distortion of the face may occur and the patients may hold onto a bedpost in absolute agony. Light touches, facial movements, chewing, talking, or drafts of air across the face precipitate the attack. There appears to be an increased frequency of attacks during episodes of fatigue or tension. Patients have such a fear of provoking an attack that they tend to immobilize themselves. According to Dr. Robert Nugent, Professor and Chairman of the Department of Neurosurgery at West Virginia University School of Medicine, "Trigeminal neuralgia is said to be the worst pain that man is heir to. It is a devastating pain that is just unbearable in its several forms" (West Virginia University Newsletter, 1986). Mild cases sometimes respond to certain medications such as carbamazepine, which prevents conduction through the nerve, but medical therapy is usually unsatisfactory. Injections, compression of the nerve, sectioning the nerve by surgery, alcoholic injection of the nerve, inhalation of trichlorethylene, electrocoagulation, radio frequency thermocoagulation, and other manipulations made on the nerve may be effective for months or years.

The two following case histories serve as excellent examples of this clinical entity. A middle-aged executive of a large manufacturing company awoke one evening with stabbing pains along the side of his face that radiated to his upper teeth with a concomitant deep burning pain just below the ear. The pain disappeared after fifteen minutes of intensive suffering, only to reappear two hours later following yawning. The pain was more severe than in the first attack. He tried heat applications, pressure with the hands, position changes, and medicating himself with six aspirin, all to no avail. His wife took him to a hospital emergency room, where an injection of Demerol abated his pain completely. A week later, following a high-pressure business meeting, a paroxysm of severe pain traversed his face like a lightning bolt, stopped abruptly, but recurred a few minutes later when the patient went out into the cool air on the way to his automobile. The pain stopped, but started again while he was driving home. This man went directly to his family physician, who sent him to a dentist. The latter found an abscessed tooth, and when he injected the involved tooth with a local anesthetic agent (to eliminate pain), the pain immediately disappeared. The tooth was subsequently extracted, and the abscess was treated with antibiotics. The patient remained pain-free thereafter.

The second case involved a middle-aged male with trigeminal neuralgia who had frequent attacks that were unresponsive to carbamazepine, and injection of the nerve with alcohol was unsuccessful. The pain was so severe that he would scream violently, holding onto a bedpost or similar object. The patient became addicted to high doses of narcotics but refused surgery to cut the nerve branch. He was found hanging from a beam in the basement accompanied by a suicide note reading, "Forgive me but I can no longer stand the pain."

EFFECTS OF THE CROWN OF THORNS

Now that we have a basic knowledge of the characteristics of the plant used to plait the crown of thorns and a brief familiarity with the anatomy of the head region, with some insight into the effects of irritating the nerves that supply pain perception to these areas, let us now examine the probable effects of the crown of thorns during the mock coronation of Christ. Scriptures relate that the soldiers filed past Jesus, taking the reed from him and striking it down on the crown of thorns. It is important to note that the crown was made by interweaving (plaiting) the thorn twigs into the shape of a cap. This placed a large number of thorns in contact with the entire top of the head, including the front, back, and sides. The blows from the reed across Jesus' face or against the thorns would directly irritate the nerves or activate trigger zones along the lip, side of the nose, or face, bringing on severe pains resembling a hot poker or electric shock lancinating across the sides of his face or deep to his ears. The pain would stop almost abruptly, only to recur again with the slightest movement of the jaws or even from a wisp of wind, stopping Jesus "dead" in his tracks. The traumatic shock from the brutal scourging would be further enhanced with each

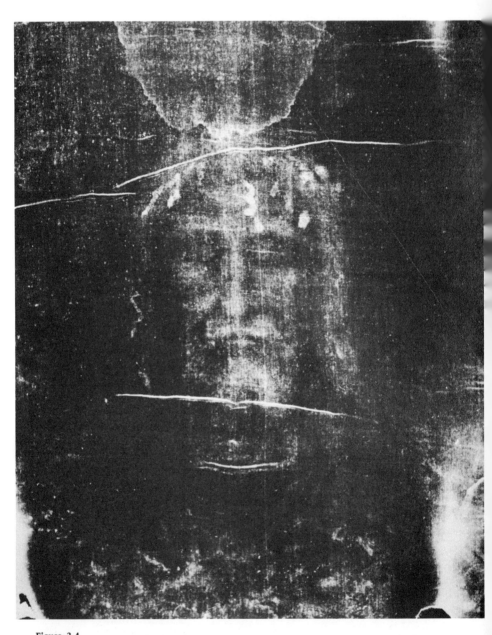

Figure 3-4
Shroud of Turin, head region.
Note the tortuous impressions (white) on the forehead, which represent blood from injuries caused by the crown of thorns.

paroxysmal pain across the face bringing him to his knees. Exacerbations and remissions of throbbing bolts of pain would occur all the way to Calvary and during crucifixion, being activated by the movements of walking, falling, and twisting, from pressure of the thorns against the cross stipes, and from the many shoves and blows by the soldiers.

Because the head region contains a plethora of blood vessels, the blood would run freely down the face. This is very dramatically depicted in the Turin Shroud, which shows images representing rivulets and seepage points running down the forehead and confirms that the crown of thorns was plaited in the shape of a cap and not a circlet (Figure 3-4). This is an important fact for Christ's crucifixion. The various blows across the face are shown on the Shroud particularly in the region of the forehead, brow, right upper lip, jaw, and nose. The tridimensional pattern more vividly reveals a broken nose and confirms the above injuries (Figure 12-16).

4
Crucifixion—Historic Aspects

HISTORIC BACKGROUND

Crucifixion was a barbaric form of capital punishment practiced by the Romans, Persians, Phoenicians, Egyptians, Greeks, Seleucids, Carthaginians, and Jews. It was most widespread prior to the birth of Christ and is believed to be a punishment of Oriental origin, although some historians think it originated in Asia Minor with the Phoenicians and Persians, who were famous for their torture techniques, which included impaling, burning in oil, drowning, beating, and crucifixion. Early sources also indicate that it was used by the Indians, Assyrians, Scythians, Taureans, Germani, and Numidians. Crucifixion was so common that during the slave uprisings led by Spartacus in B.C. 73–71, about six thousand crosses lined the road from Rome to Capua. Although crucifixion was abolished by Emperor Constantine in the fourth century, Professor Paola Ricca relates that a recent paper by Professor Angelo Gramaglia of the Turin Seminary has shown that in the seventh century, during the fighting between the Arabs and Christians, there were mass crucifixions of Christians in the manner that Jesus was crucified, as a sign of contempt.

Crucifixion is derived from the word *cruciare*, to torture and torment, and was an ignominious fate reserved for traitors, slaves, hardened murderers, political or religious agitators, pirates, and individuals who had no rights. Historical sources indicate that in B.C. 519, Darius I, the Persian king, had three thousand political opponents crucified; Antiochus IV of Syria had Jews in Jerusalem flogged and crucified for breaking laws; Alexander Jannaeus, the Judean king, had eight hundred opponents crucified in B.C. 88 after Herod's death; and Publius Quintilius Varus had two thousand crucified. According to the historian Flavius Josephus, about five hundred Jewish prisoners were crucified per day under the Emperor Titus in 70 A.D., during the siege of Jerusalem.

It appears that the Romans learned the technique of crucifixion from the Carthaginians. Cicero, in the first century B.C., referred to crucifixion as "the most cruel and atrocious of punishments" (*Crudelissimum eterrimumque supplicum*). It was a supreme deterrent against political and military crimes and very effective in maintaining law and order. Even though Cicero felt that no Roman citizen could be crucified, in many instances of high treason or serious crimes against the state, they were punished by this method.

THE ROMAN METHOD

It may be of interest that the Romans considered crucifixion a deterrent to crime. It was reserved at that time primarily for provincials, criminals, and slaves (*servile supplicum*) and was initiated methodically with utmost precision. Every Roman soldier was well trained in every step of the technique.

THE EXECUTIONERS

The *exactor mortis*, a centurion, was in charge of four Roman soldiers, called the *quaternio*, who were entrusted with the duty of crucifixion. They were expert in the art of crucifixion and completed their task with utmost facility. Because crucifixions were very common, the execution team did not lack experience. The entire procedure was effected with great dispatch because of their vast experience. The *exactor mortis* was also entrusted with the responsibility of determining if the victim was dead and reporting this to the procurator, who then officially filed a certification. The Roman soldiers were also expert in making this determination because crucifixion was an almost daily occurrence.

5

The Cross, the Nails, and the Title

THE CROSS

Throughout the period when crucifixion was practiced, several kinds of crosses were used. The basic forms were the *crux simplex*, composed of a single stake to which the hands were fastened above the head and the feet were fastened below (*affixio*), and the *crux compacta*, which consisted of two parts, the upright referred to as the *stipes* or *staticulum*, and the crosspiece, called the *patibulum* or *antenna*. The *crux compacta* varied in one of the following three forms. The *crux commissa* resembled the capital letter T and was sometimes referred to as the T-cross. The *crux immissa*, or *capitata*, is the conventional cross usually displayed in churches and sometimes called the Roman cross; its *stipes* projected above the *patibulum* (Figure 5-1). This form is the one that most scholars believe was used to crucify Jesus because Scriptures relate that the *titulus* or title (placard) was placed above his head depicting the nature of his crime. "Jesus of Nazareth, the King of the Jews" (Mark 15:26 and John 19:19). This, of course, depended in a large degree on the width of the *patibulum* because experiments reveal sufficient space even on the *crux commissa*. Another form, the *crux decussata* or X-cross, was also referred to as the Cross of St. Andrew because this was the form used to crucify St. Andrew at Patrae. This form may not have been unique to St. Andrew because the historian Josephus, in the *Jewish War*, reports that during the

32

siege of Jerusalem, the Romans crucified Jews in a multiplicity of positions.

THE CRUCIFIXION SITE

The *stipes* or *staticulum* were constructed of strong wood and were usually permanently fixed in the ground in a hilly area on the city's outskirts just beyond the walls so that the crucified were conspicuously displayed in full view. In Rome, crucifixion was initiated in the Esquiline Camp, just outside of the Servian walls, where the vulturelike birds of the Esquiline awaited their prey—the bodies of the crucified. The same pattern was true in Jerusalem. The Romans set up their place of execution just outside the walls, in a hilly, conspicuous region called Calvary (Latin: *calvarii*) or Golgotha (Aramaic: *Gulgutha*), both of which mean "skull," probably because of the shape of this hilly knoll. It is of interest that the place of crucifixion was close to the nearby tombs.

HEIGHT OF THE CROSS

There have been differences of opinion as to the height of the *staticulum* because historical references allude to both high and low

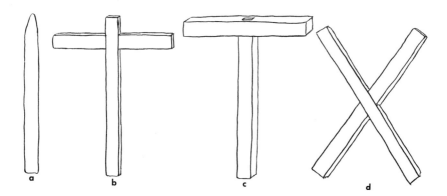

Figure 5-1

Types of crosses.
(a) crux simplex *(simple stake).*
(b) crux immissa or capitata *(conventional).*
(c) crux commissa *(T cross).*
(d) crux decussata *(Cross of St. Andrew). The* crux compacta *included types b, c, and d and was composed of two parts, the upright called the* stipes *or* staticulum *and the crosspiece called the* patibulum.

crosses. The former, among the Romans, was reserved primarily for special criminals who in some way had caused dishonor to a Roman. In general, however, the Roman crosses probably stood about seven to seven and a half feet in height because, from a practical point of view, it was easier to lift the crosspiece (*patibulum*) into position on a shorter cross after nailing the upper extremities of the victim to it. Conversely, it was easier to remove the victim from the cross after death. The shorter crosses also made it easier for wild animals to finish off victims. This contention is also supported by the fact that a short reed (hyssop) (Mark 15:36) was used to bring the *posca* to his lips. If the *patibulum* was about seven to seven and a half feet, an individual who was about 5′4″ tall (estimated average height of a man of that era) would need to utilize a reed from the hyssop plant measuring about eighteen inches to two feet long. The height is also compatible with the wound on the right side of the Shroud of Turin for the correct angle of penetration into the heart or pericardial sac by the spear.

THE SADDLE

There was much controversy as to whether the upright contained a saddle (*sedile, pegma, cornu, horn*) about halfway up the cross that protruded, according to Cicero, like a rhinoceros's horn. The victim was straddled to it to support the body periodically in order to ease his misery (*equitar cruci*, to ride a cross). It has been charged by many workers that a *sedile* was necessary because the victim would not be able to survive for very long periods without this support and the nails through the hands would have surely pulled through. It is difficult, however, to conceive how a *sedile* could be permanently placed on a cross that would satisfy the height of all individuals, particularly in relation to the nailing of the hands. Our experiments show that the angle of the arms on the *patibulum* varies from sixty to seventy degrees according to an individual's structural variations. Our experiments also show that when the feet are bound to the cross (or nailed) there is little need for body support. This is also true of the *suppedaneum* (support) that many investigators indicate would be required for much the same reason. This question will be elaborated on more fully in a subsequent section. The *sedile*, however, was usually used when it was desired to have a crucified individual remain on the cross for long periods of time, sometimes for many days. For example,

Lipsius tells of two cases where victims hung for nine days, but this appears difficult to believe, particularly if the hands and feet were nailed. Perhaps, if the hands and feet were bound by ropes alone and the victim was not scourged beforehand, this might be possible. It must also be remembered that the weekend of Christ's crucifixion was an unusually sacrosanct one. It fell on a double religious holiday, the Passover and the Sabbath. Therefore, it would be highly unlikely that any means to prolong his life would have been allowed, because sundown would soon be at hand.

KIND OF WOOD

The type of wood that crosses were made of was variable, usually depending on the wood available. It was hewn very roughly. Micropaleobotanical studies of fragments of alleged relics of the true cross reveal that it was made of pine. The most definitive study, however, was made on the piece of wood found on the end of the nail discovered in the heel bones of a crucified man that was excavated in the Jewish Quarter of the Old City of Jerusalem in 1969–70 and dated to about A.D. 7. The paleobotanical study of this piece of wood revealed it to be from the olive tree (Figure 5-2). However, this could not be confirmed by a botanist from the Hebrew University of Jerusalem using a scanning electron microscope, as the sample was too minute. Although Yaden contended that it was unlikely that olive wood was used for the upright of the cross because the trunk and branches are bent and crooked, it cannot be discounted because on occasion they attain a height of two to three meters.

LEGENDS OF THE CROSS

It is of only passing interest that legends on the origin of the wood are legion, but I am including a few for the reader's interest. In Germany, the legend states that the pear tree took root and bloomed with flowers of a blood-red color after the death of Christ. In the United States, it is said that the flowery petals of the beautiful dogwood tree are stained red and drawn in as a reminder of Christ's wounds. In Poland, they attribute the cross to the aspen, which contained leaves that tremble in fear of God's vengeance. Another legend relates that the aspen tree will protect one against lightning, whereas the poplar trees, which are related to aspens,

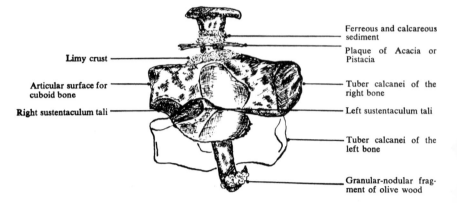

Ferreous and calcareous sediment

Plaque of Acacia or Pistacia

Limy crust

Articular surface for cuboid bone

Right sustentaculum tali

Tuber calcanei of the right bone

Left sustentaculum tali

Tuber calcanei of the left bone

Granular-nodular fragment of olive wood

Figure 5-2
Diagram of the heel bone of a crucified man from A.D. 7.
The nail is still present and bent at the tip, which contains a piece of wood believed to be olive wood. A plaque under the head of the nail also contains wood. From the excavations of the Tombs of Giv'at ha Mivtar in the Jewish Quarter of Jerusalem. (Courtesy of the Israel Exploration Society and Mrs. Nicu Haas.)

will not afford this protection. A legend in England indicates that the mistletoe was used to make the cross, and ever since, it has been relegated to the status of a humble parasite. Similarly, in Italy, the clematis was considered the source of the cross, and the story has it that at the time of crucifixion it was a large tree condemned forever to be a low-growing vine. In other countries, the oak, the alder, and the pine have been implicated. In this regard, it is believed that the pine started producing crosslike whorls after the crucifixion.

THE NAILS

The nails used in crucifixion at the time of Christ bear little resemblance to the nails that we conventionally use in carpentry. The Roman nails were made of iron with a gradually tapering square shaft from head to point. About ten years ago, seven tons of homemade nails (almost a million nails) were unearthed in Scotland by Professor I. A. Richmond, Professor of Archaeology of the Roman Empire at Oxford, at the site of a Roman fortress at Inchtuthill, built in A.D. 83. These nails ranged from about 1 to 40 centimeters long (Figure 5-3).

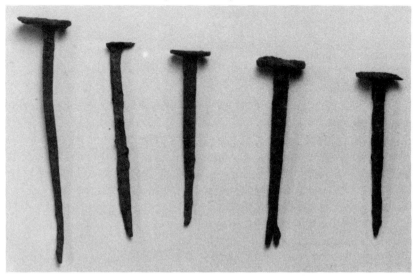

Figure 5-3
Roman nails ca. A.D. 83.
Seven tons of homemade iron nails from the site of a Roman fortress at Inchtuthill, Scotland.
(Courtesy of Sir Geoffrey Ford, The Institute of Metals, London.)

A relic of great interest now on exhibit in the Basilica of S. Croce in Gerusalemme, in Rome, Italy, was allegedly found by Helen, mother of the Emperor Constantine, near the beginning of the third century, and is purported to be one of the nails used in the crucifixion of Jesus. The nail is 12.5 centimeters long, has a square iron shaft that measures 9 millimeters at the head and tapers gradually to the point area, where it measures 5 millimeters. The head of the nail is in the shape of a dome with the edges extended as in a bell. A nail similar to this has been constructed for experimental purposes and is depicted in Figure 5-4. It is of interest to note that this nail bears a strong resemblance to the nail recovered from the Giv'at ha Mivtar excavation (Figure 7-17). The latter is about 12 centimeters long but was probably slightly longer in its original state.

THE TITLE

Pilate also wrote a title and put it on the cross. It read, "Jesus of Nazareth, the King of the Jews." Many of the Jews read this title,

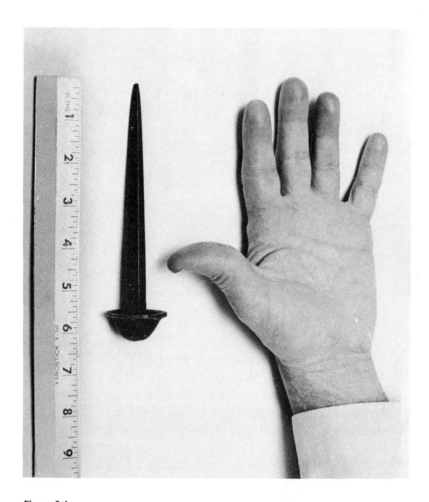

Figure 5-4
Iron nail sized against a human hand.
Replica of the nail on display in the Chapel of Gerusalemme in Rome. Found in the third century by St. Helen and believed to be one of the nails that was used to crucify Jesus.

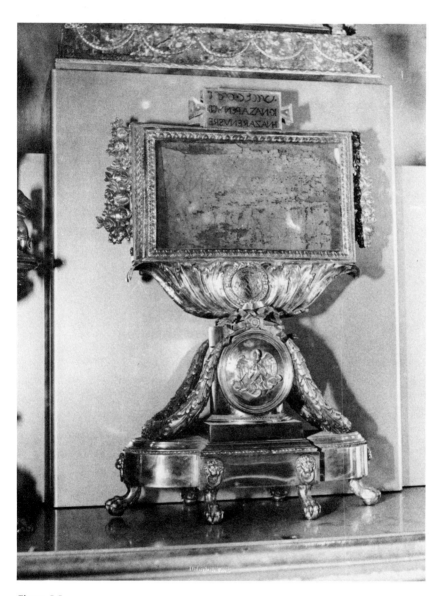

Figure 5-5
Relic of deteriorated titulus.
Also found in the third century by St. Helen and on display in the Holy Chapel of Gerusalemme. Believed to be the titulus on the cross that Jesus was crucified on. The characters appear in Aramaic, Greek and Latin.

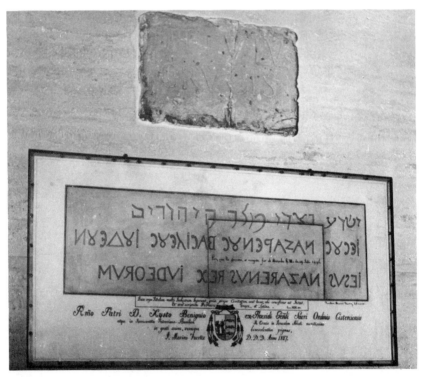

Figure 5-6
Reconstruction of the titulus from the relic as depicted in the previous illustration.

for the place where Jesus was crucified was near the city; and it was written in Hebrew, in Latin and in Greek (John 19:19–20). "Over his head they put the charges against him which read, 'This is Jesus, King of the Jews'" (Matthew 27:37).

The *titulus* (title) was the piece of tablet containing the crime of the *cruciarius* (victim) and was usually nailed to the cross above the victim's head. This was carried by the condemned individual, usually around his neck, from the place of sentencing and was part of the parade all the way to the crucifixion site.

The chief priest made much of the fact that Christ's crime was written as being King of the Jews and objected vehemently to Pilate, "Do not write 'King of the Jews,' but, 'This man said, I am King of the Jews,'" but Pilate answered him, "What I have written,

I have written" (John 19:21–22). It appears that Pilate was no longer worried about the previous pressures about reportimg him to Rome. The above quoted scriptural references that the *titulus* was nailed above his head is the single most important argument that the *crux immissa* was used rather than the *crux commissa*. Our experiments indicate, however, that there was enough room for the title on the *crux commissa*. This is hardly important because the degree and type of suffering exhibited by Christ would be identical, regardless of which of the two crosses was used.

The Basilica of S. Croce in Gerusalemme also contains a relic purported to be a part of the *titulus* containing characters in Latin, Greek, and Hebrew or Syro-Chaldaic. This badly deteriorated relic was allegedly found in Jerusalem by St. Helen in the early third century (Figure 5-5). A full proportional reproduction of the title was made using the relic piece as a base (Figure 5-6), and the characters are written from right to left. The inscription of the victim's crime in three languages, related only by St. John, was probably done routinely because in *Jewish War*, Volume 5.2, Josephus, the historian, indicates that slabs placed at various intervals bore warnings, some written in Latin and some in Greek. The biographer Julius Capitolinus wrote in the fourth century of a title written in Greek, Aramaic, Egyptian, and Persian and placed over the sepulcher of the murdered emperor Giorgianus Pius. Moreover, the *Interpreter's Bible* indicates that there was a need for the three languages in Jerusalem because Latin was the official administrative language, Aramaic was spoken by the Jews of the time, and Greek was the language of international commerce and culture.

6

The Way to the Skull

"**T**hen he handed Him over to them to be crucified. So they took Jesus, and He went out, bearing His own cross to the place called the Place of the Skull, which is called in Hebrew, Golgotha" (John 19:16–17).

CARRYING THE CROSS

It was about noon, and the trip from Antonia to Golgotha (Calvary) was along one of the main streets and measured over one-half mile (Figure 6-1). It was an unpaved, bumpy road studded with scores of crevices made by the carts and beasts of burden. As one approached the outside walls, the road assumed an uphill climb. The weather at that time was hot and dry, and Jesus, the *cruciarius*, was paraded through the main street, carrying the crosspiece weighing about fifty pounds, balanced across one or both shoulders (Figure 6-2). He also carried the *titulus* (title) or piece of tablet around his neck naming the crime he was accused of, which would subsequently be nailed above his head on the cross. The *exactor mortis* and his team of four escorted Jesus while numerous soldiers lined the street to maintain order and to quell any riots because a serried mass of hostile people lined the streets, spitting and cursing at him as he passed by.

It is important to evaluate Christ's medical condition in order to understand the full impact of his sufferings and agony. At this time, he was in a state of extreme exhaustion resulting from the

42

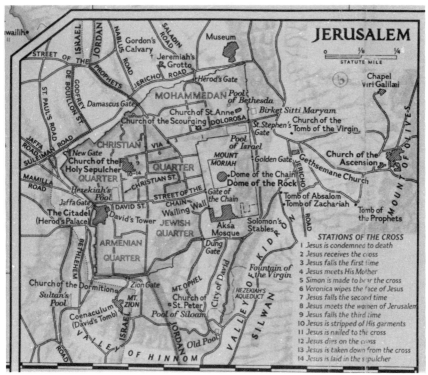

Figure 6-1
Map of the Jerusalem area showing the cross on the road to Calvary.
This trek measures over a half mile.

severe mental sufferings endured at the Garden of Gethsemane, which included a physical loss of sweat and blood, the brutal flogging at the praetorium, and the nerve-racking, lancinating pains from the crown of thorns. It is safe to assume that Jesus was already in a state of traumatic shock. The intense heat of the sun and the weight of the *patibulum* on his lacerated shoulders would induce intense weakness and dizziness or lightheadedness, causing him to stumble, totter, and fall. The noon sun was high, and the sweat poured over him (the Franciscan Way of the Cross depicts Jesus falling three times). This contention is not compatible with his clinical status. When we consider his condition, there is little doubt that Christ fell many times before arriving at Calvary. It was the *exactor mortis's* responsibility to make certain that the *cruciarius*

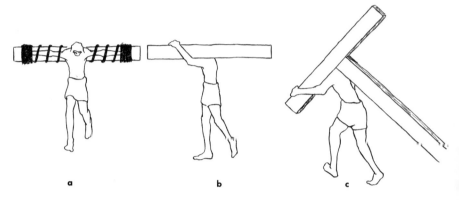

Figure 6-2

Carrying the cross.
(a) The arms are tied to the patibulum with ropes.
(b) The patibulum is balanced on one shoulder.
(c) The way the entire cross would be carried.

would get his just punishment of crucifixion and not die on the way. The *exactor mortis* was fearful that Jesus might not get up again and that he would not be able to execute his orders. He therefore delegated Simon of Cyrene, a passerby, to carry the *patibulum* for Jesus. Before Simon carried the cross, every time Jesus tripped and fell, lancinating pains would radiate across his face and scalp and precipitate severe pains in all of his muscles and joints. He had more and more difficulty getting up each time he fell while bearing the weight of the cross. As a physician, I find it almost incredible that he was able to make the trek to Calvary at all. He certainly had to be highly motivated.

Most scholars support the concept that only the crosspiece or *patibulum* was usually carried by the *cruciarius* to the place of crucifixion. This issue has not been definitively decided because scientists such as Barbet estimated the weight of the cross to be about 220 pounds, with the crosspiece weighing about 110 pounds. They felt that this would be too heavy to carry. Innitzer's group, however, estimates that the entire cross weighed only about 95–128 pounds, with the crossbeam weighing only about 36–48 pounds. Consultation with experienced builders who work with lumber on a daily basis indicates to me that a heavy 8–9-foot oak beam with a 6-

foot crosspiece would weigh only about 125–130 pounds, with the crosspiece weighing about 50–55 pounds. The cumbersome cross would invariably have to be dragged by the victim in a slumped position with one arm of the cross being placed on the shoulder (Figure 6-2). Moreover, the large number of *stipes* (the uprights) already standing outside the city's wall adds greater support to the concept that he carried only the crosspiece.

There are two schools of thought regarding the manner in which the crosspiece was carried. Most scholars embrace the con-cept that each end of the crosspiece was tied to the victim's wrists and arms (Figure 6-2), but the cross might have been balanced on one shoulder. The latter concept would be compatible with the statement of Tertullian that Jesus carried his cross on his shoulder. Some authors interpreted this as being the whole cross because they were under the impression that the *patibulum* had to be carried on both shoulders. In Jesus' case, it would have been a difficult task to remove the ties from each wrist, to remove the *patibulum* and then place it on Simon of Cyrene's shoulders, and again tie the wrists securely. Sindologists interpret two images on the back of the Shroud of Turin as evidence that the cross was placed over both shoulders and tied to the wrists. This interpretation, however, is subject to debate, and the reader is referred to Chapter 12 for additional information.

JESUS ARRIVES AT CALVARY

When Jesus arrived at the crucifixion site, he was almost numb with exhaustion accompanied by marked shortness of breath because fluid had accumulated within and around his lungs as a consequence of the brutal scourging. His clothing was literally glued to his body by the blood in the open flagellation wounds, which had clotted to his vesture. In the Roman mode, the clothing was usually removed following scourging, but because of the Jewish sensitivities, the robe obviously was left on Jesus during the journey to Calvary. Scriptures tell us that the soldiers cast lots for his garments (Mark 15:24), probably because the tunic was unsewn and completely woven in one piece making it too valuable to tear into four pieces. The dice were rolled, and it was the winner's job to remove the victim's vesture, for it now belonged to him. I wonder how he accomplished this feat. Did he soak the garments to soften the blood clots, as we physicians and nurses do frequently when removing a bandage that has adhered firmly to a wound? If one remembers that the name of the game was pain, then the mode is clear. It was unquestionably yanked off, sending jolts of pain throughout his body. Everyone remembers having a sibling or friend who related that the easy way to remove a bandage that is adherent to a wound is to yank it off quickly. Even though the pain was only momentary, think of how many of these sharp pains you would experience if a giant gauze pad was stuck to the front and back of your whole body, including your arms, and it was suddenly pulled off. Here was Jesus of Nazareth, King of the Jews, lying naked on the ground in a state of utter exhaustion, his body racked with pain, and still to face the most ignominious of suffering, the terrifying crucifixion.

7

Nailing of the Hands and Feet

NAILING OF THE HANDS

When Jesus appeared to his disciples and showed them his hands and feet, he said "See my hands and my feet, that it is myself" (Luke 24:39), and "He showed them his hands and side. . . ." Then he said to Thomas, "Put your finger here, and see my hands; and put out your hand, and place it in my side. . . ." (John 20:20–27). Moreover, Psalm 22:16, which is believed to have predicted the Messiah's fate, relates, "they pierced my hands and my feet."

One of the major controversies in sindonology concerns the anatomical location of the hand wound when Jesus was nailed to the *patibulum* (crosspiece) of the cross. For centuries, most devout Christians believed that the nails passed through the palms of the hands in accord with the scriptural texts quoted above. Even ancient historians like Lipsius related that it was the hands that were transfixed in crucifixion, and early crucifixes, such as the ivory crucifix, dated to A.D. 420 in the British Museum (Figure 7-1), and the crucifix on a wooden portal of S. Sabena in Rome, dated to the first half of the fifth century, showed the nails through the center of the palms. Everything was peaceful until the 1932 Exposition of the Shroud of Turin when Dr. Pierre Barbet, a Parisian surgeon, expounded the hypothesis that the palm of the hand could not support the weight of the body and that the nail actually passed through the wrist emerging at a focus corresponding

47

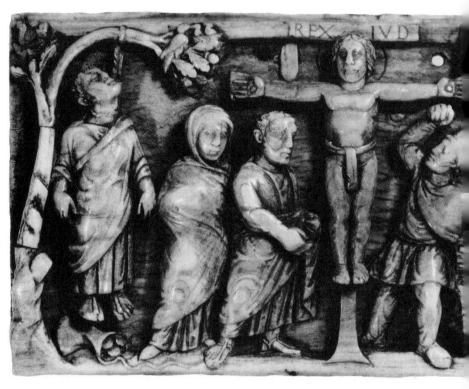

Figure 7-1
Christ crucified and Judas hanging.
Ivory, casket panel, ca. 420 A.D., British Museum.
Courtesy of the Trustees of the British Museum.

to where the image of the hand wound is located on the Shroud of Turin. His conclusions were based on hand anatomy, on observations made by artists who had hung cadavers to the cross, and on his personal experiments. He further supported his hypothesis by so reverently quoting from the revelations of St. Brigit, "My son's hands were pierced at the spot where the bone was most solid." However, when he developed his hypothesis that one nail pierced both feet, he totally ignored St. Brigit's revelation that each foot was pierced separately.

Barbet's hypothesis is so entrenched in Shroud and crucifixion research that it is almost completely accepted as factual and has been quoted in articles and books, *ad infinitum*. Yet, no valid experimental studies to confirm or refute his hypothesis had ever been conducted prior to my own studies.

The unfortunate thing about this whole state of affairs is that *there are serious errors in Barbet's hypothesis that make his hypothesis totally untenable.* Before investigating the source of these errors, it is important that we briefly review the essential features of the anatomy of the hand and forearm and the mechanical principles regarding the amount of pull exerted on each hand during suspension on the cross.

ANATOMY OF THE HAND

Let us briefly review the essential features of the anatomy of the hand and forearm basic to an understanding of its structural integrity in relation to its fixation to the cross. It is important during this discussion that you constantly refer to the diagrams indicated. The palm of the hand is the front of the hand and does not include the fingers and thumb. This area contains a triangular fibrous structure called the palmar aponeurosis with the greater bulk of the fibers in parallel bands and with some transverse fibers running perpendicular to these bands (Figure 7-2). Although the transverse fibers may offer some support, the parallel fibers would offer little or no support if a nail were passed through this region. Another supportive structure, at the base of the fingers, is the superficial transverse metacarpal ligaments. The skin of the palm is thick and bound tightly to the palmar aponeurosis, in contrast to the *dorsum* (back) of the hand, where the skin is loose and pliable. There are, however, fibers from the deep muscles and tendons on the back of the hand that provide strength and structural integrity.

Now open your hand and observe the bulky prominence extending into the hand from the base of the thumb to the wrist. This is called the thenar eminence (Figure 7-2). If you touch the tip of your thumb to the tip of your little finger, you will note a deep furrow at the base of the thenar eminence called the thenar furrow. A branch of the median nerve coming from the wrist runs in this furrow. The wrist or carpus is composed of eight small bones, depicted in Figures 7-3 and 7-4, tightly bound to each other by interlacing ligaments that afford strength to this area.

The region at the end of the bones of the forearm (radius and ulna) is extremely strong because the ends of the two bones abut against each other and are entwined by strong ligaments. More-

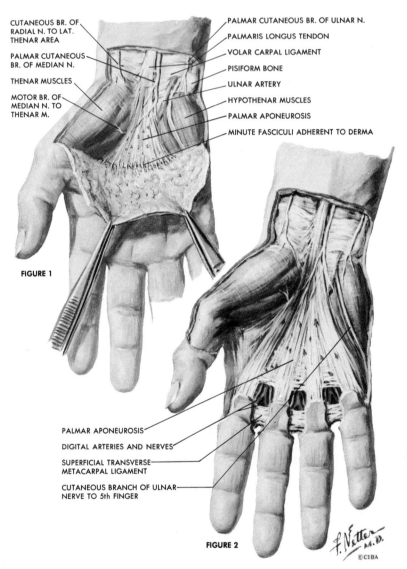

CUTANEOUS BR. OF RADIAL N. TO LAT. THENAR AREA

PALMAR CUTANEOUS BR. OF MEDIAN N.

THENAR MUSCLES

MOTOR BR. OF MEDIAN N. TO THENAR M.

PALMAR CUTANEOUS BR. OF ULNAR N.

PALMARIS LONGUS TENDON

VOLAR CARPAL LIGAMENT

PISIFORM BONE

ULNAR ARTERY

HYPOTHENAR MUSCLES

PALMAR APONEUROSIS

MINUTE FASCICULI ADHERENT TO DERMA

FIGURE 1

PALMAR APONEUROSIS

DIGITAL ARTERIES AND NERVES

SUPERFICIAL TRANSVERSE METACARPAL LIGAMENT

CUTANEOUS BRANCH OF ULNAR NERVE TO 5th FINGER

FIGURE 2

REG. NO. 675

Figure 7-2

Palm of the hand.

Note the palmar aponeurosis (triangular fibrous structure), the transverse metacar-pal ligament at the base of the fingers, the thenar eminence (muscle) and the palmaris longus tendon. The median nerve runs from the wrist along the thenar furrow.
(Illustration by Frank Netter, from Clinical Symposia. *Courtesy of Ciba Phar-maceutical Co., copyright 1957.)*

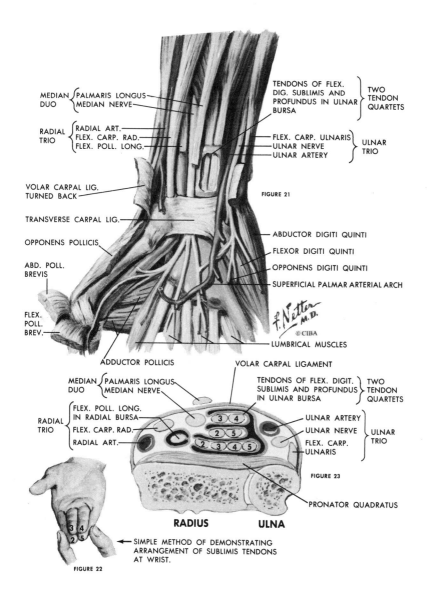

MEDIAN {PALMARIS LONGUS
DUO   {MEDIAN NERVE

RADIAL {RADIAL ART.
TRIO   {FLEX. CARP. RAD.
       {FLEX. POLL. LONG.

VOLAR CARPAL LIG.
TURNED BACK

TRANSVERSE CARPAL LIG.

OPPONENS POLLICIS

ABD. POLL.
BREVIS

FLEX.
POLL.
BREV.

ADDUCTOR POLLICIS

TENDONS OF FLEX.
DIG. SUBLIMIS AND   } TWO
PROFUNDUS IN ULNAR   } TENDON
BURSA   } QUARTETS

FLEX. CARP. ULNARIS }
ULNAR NERVE   } ULNAR
ULNAR ARTERY   } TRIO

FIGURE 21

ABDUCTOR DIGITI QUINTI

FLEXOR DIGITI QUINTI

OPPONENS DIGITI QUINTI

SUPERFICIAL PALMAR ARTERIAL ARCH

LUMBRICAL MUSCLES

©CIBA

MEDIAN {PALMARIS LONGUS
DUO   {MEDIAN NERVE

RADIAL {FLEX. POLL. LONG.
TRIO   {IN RADIAL BURSA
       {FLEX. CARP. RAD.
       {RADIAL ART.

VOLAR CARPAL LIGAMENT

TENDONS OF FLEX. DIGIT. } TWO
SUBLIMIS AND PROFUNDUS } TENDON
IN ULNAR BURSA   } QUARTETS

ULNAR ARTERY }
ULNAR NERVE   } ULNAR
FLEX. CARP.   } TRIO
ULNARIS

FIGURE 23

PRONATOR QUADRATUS

RADIUS   ULNA

SIMPLE METHOD OF DEMONSTRATING
ARRANGEMENT OF SUBLIMIS TENDONS
AT WRIST.

FIGURE 22

Figure 7-3

Hand and wrist.

Anatomy of the deeper layers of the hand showing the eight small bones of the wrist and the median nerve and its branches. The nail would pass through the Z-area formed by the capitate, lesser multangular and two metacarpal bones of the index and second finger. This is a very sturdy region (see text).
(Illustration by Frank Netter, from Clinical Symposia. *Courtesy of Ciba Pharmaceutical Co., copyright 1957.)*

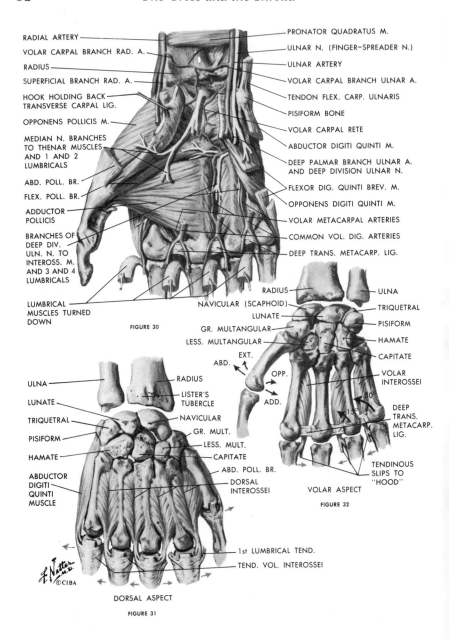

RADIAL ARTERY
VOLAR CARPAL BRANCH RAD. A.
RADIUS
SUPERFICIAL BRANCH RAD. A.
HOOK HOLDING BACK TRANSVERSE CARPAL LIG.
OPPONENS POLLICIS M.
MEDIAN N. BRANCHES TO THENAR MUSCLES AND 1 AND 2 LUMBRICALS
ABD. POLL. BR.
FLEX. POLL. BR.
ADDUCTOR POLLICIS
BRANCHES OF DEEP DIV. ULN. N. TO INTEROSS. M. AND 3 AND 4 LUMBRICALS
LUMBRICAL MUSCLES TURNED DOWN

PRONATOR QUADRATUS M.
ULNAR N. (FINGER–SPREADER N.)
ULNAR ARTERY
VOLAR CARPAL BRANCH ULNAR A.
TENDON FLEX. CARP. ULNARIS
PISIFORM BONE
VOLAR CARPAL RETE
ABDUCTOR DIGITI QUINTI M.
DEEP PALMAR BRANCH ULNAR A. AND DEEP DIVISION ULNAR N.
FLEXOR DIG. QUINTI BREV. M.
OPPONENS DIGITI QUINTI M.
VOLAR METACARPAL ARTERIES
COMMON VOL. DIG. ARTERIES
DEEP TRANS. METACARP. LIG.

FIGURE 30

RADIUS
NAVICULAR (SCAPHOID)
LUNATE
GR. MULTANGULAR
LESS. MULTANGULAR
EXT.
ABD.
OPP.
ADD.

ULNA
TRIQUETRAL
PISIFORM
HAMATE
CAPITATE
VOLAR INTEROSSEI
DEEP TRANS. METACARP. LIG.
TENDINOUS SLIPS TO "HOOD"
VOLAR ASPECT

FIGURE 32

ULNA
LUNATE
TRIQUETRAL
PISIFORM
HAMATE
ABDUCTOR DIGITI QUINTI MUSCLE

RADIUS
LISTER'S TUBERCLE
NAVICULAR
GR. MULT.
LESS. MULT.
CAPITATE
ABD. POLL. BR.
DORSAL INTEROSSEI

1st LUMBRICAL TEND.
TEND. VOL. INTEROSSEI

DORSAL ASPECT

FIGURE 31

Figure 7-4
Hand and wrist.
Branches of the median nerve and the palmaris longus tendon. Note that the median nerve runs on the thumb side of this tendon.
(Illustration by Frank Netter, from Clinical Symposia. *Courtesy of Ciba Pharmaceutical Co., copyright 1957.)*

over, the strength of both the carpus region and other structures above renders additional reinforcement to this area.

THE AMOUNT OF PULL ON EACH HAND

It is important to realize that if the point of the nail was directed slightly upward, it would pass between the metacarpal bones, which would be unable to support the weight of the body without reinforcement with ropes. This is obviously the region of the palm that is the center of the controversy. The *exactor mortis* and his team would certainly have been aware through their training and their experience in crucifying hundreds of victims that if the nails were driven too high on the palms, additional support with ropes would be necessary. The weakness of this region was confirmed by Barbet's experiment, when he nailed the hands of freshly amputated arms and suspended weights on the opposite ends of them. He found that the nail tore through the hand, emerging between the fingers, when the weight of about eighty-eight pounds was added with concomitant jerking of the arm. This is important because mathematical computations indicate that there is a pull on the hands in excess of the weight of the body, and the amount of this pull was a function of the angle of the arms with the upright of the cross. For example, the pull on the arms of a suspended individual can be calculated mathematically by determining the force of tension (P) as a function of the angle the arms make with the vertical. In Figures 7-5 and 7-6, P represents the pull or tension on the arm, W is the weight of the body, and X is equilibrium. Therefore, $P \cos 0 + P \cos 0 - W = P$ or $\dfrac{W}{2 \cos 0}$.

When the arms are suspended directly above the head, there is an equal distribution of exactly one-half the weight of the body on each arm because there is only a vertical vectoral force. The greater the angle the arms create with the vertical, the greater the pull or tension on each arm because a horizontal vector or force comes into play proportional to the increase in angle. If an individual weighs 175 pounds and the arms are at a sixty-five degree angle with the vertical, the formula would be:

$$P = \frac{175}{2 \cos 0} = 87.5 \frac{1}{\cos 50} = 87.5 \frac{1}{.4227} = 207 \text{ lbs.}$$

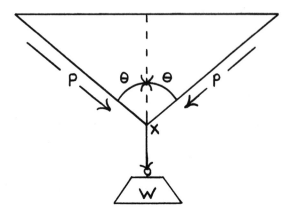

Figure 7-5
Mathematical representation of force of tension as a function of the angle the arms make with the vertical.
Pull on each hand is equal to twice the cosine of this angle.

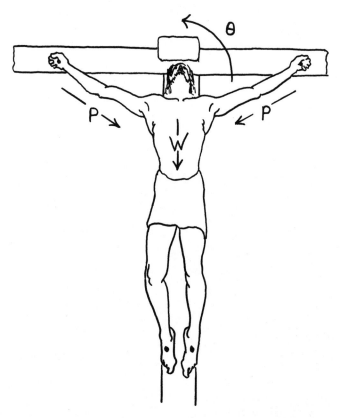

Figure 7-6
The force of tension on the arms and hands of a crucified person.

The following table shows the effects of modifying the angle of an individual weighing 175 pounds. Note that at the angle of crucifixion, which we have determined experimentally to be between sixty and seventy degrees because of individual variation, there is a pull of between 175 and 256 pounds on each arm, which is greater than the weight of the body. Note that at sixty degrees, the pull on each arm equals the full weight of the body.

TABLE 7-1
FORCE OF TENSION ON ARMS

Angle of arm with vertical	Pull on each hand in pounds
0	87.5
10	89.0
20	93.1
30	101
40	114
45	124
50	136
55	153
60	175
65	207
70	256
75	338
80	504
83	718
85	1006
87	1685
88	2500
89	4860

Tension in pounds exerted on each hand of an individual weighing 175 pounds according to the angle of each arm with the vertical.

This description may have evaded many of my readers, but for those of you who are not mathematically inclined, the following simple demonstration is self-explanatory. In Figure 7-7, a weight is suspended by two rubber bands having equal characteristics of elasticity, thickness, length, and strength. When the rubber bands are in a vertical position, each band supports half of the weight. The entire weight is suspended on just one band in Figure 7-8. The length of the band is longer than either of the two depicted in the previous diagrams, as one would expect. But note in Figure 7-9 which corresponds to the angle of suspension, each rubber band is longer than the single band that held the entire weight in Figure 7-8.

Figures 7-7–7-9

Experiments to demonstrate the amount of pull on the arms during suspension.

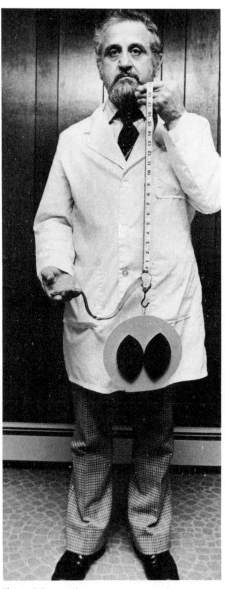 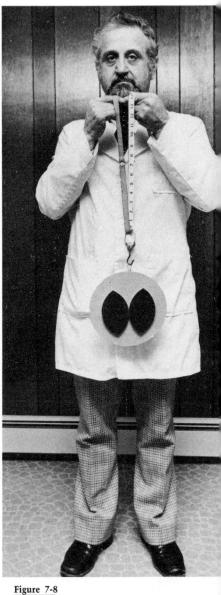

Figure 7-7
The weight is suspended by two rubber bands (one is hidden by the tape measure). The bands stretch to 14 inches each.

Figure 7-8
The entire weight is suspended by only on rubber band. The single band stretches to inches.

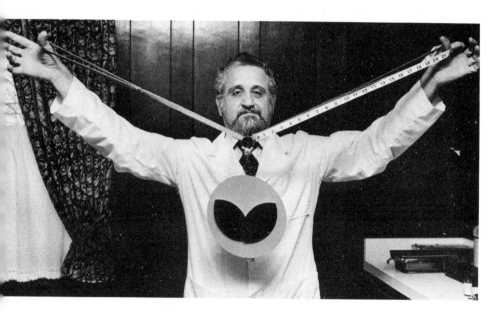

Figure 7-9

The weight is suspended by both rubber bands using the average angle of suspension on the cross. Note that the rubber bands stretch to 22 inches, which is significantly longer than in the previous figure, where the entire weight was suspended by only one rubber band.

WHY DESTOT'S SPACE HYPOTHESIS IS TOTALLY INVALID

Following the experiments discussed above, with the amputated arms, Barbet looked for a stronger area. He noted that the hand wound on the Shroud appeared to be located in the wrist area so he performed some experiments in which he passed square nails, with sides measuring one third of an inch, through the wrist and reported that the nails always found a natural path through an anatomical area called *Destot's space*. Barbet defined the location of *Destot's space* when he related ". . . one finds that in the middle of the bones of the wrists there is a free space bounded by the *capitate*, the *semilunar*, the *triquetral* and the *hamate* bones. We know this space so well that we know in accordance with Destot's work. . ." Later in defining the passage of the nail, he relates, "The nail has entered into *Destot's space*. . ."

Now that we have set the stage, where are the serious errors in his famous Destot's space hypothesis? The first major error is in the location of the hand wound on the Shroud in relation to the location of Destot's space. *The error derives from the fact that the hand wound image on the Shroud is on the radial (thumb) side of the wrist (Figure 8-2) and Destot's space is on the ulnar (little finger) side of the wrist* (Figures 7-10, 7-11, 7-12). When I first noted this, I thought that perhaps the space might angle toward the site depicted on the Shroud and emerge at this point, but upon checking I found that there was no way such a communication could be made short of fracturing bones. Then I thought that perhaps Barbet had only made an error in identifying the carpal bones of the wrist since the term Destot's space is not generally known outside of France. Then I found this was not the case because Barbet removed all doubt by providing an anatomical diagram to show Destot's space in his 1937 book, *Les cinq plaies du Christ* (Figure 7-10) but did not provide a diagram in *A Doctor at Calvary*. If you examine the position of this space on Barbet's diagram (Figure 7-10), you will find that it is on the *ulnar* (little finger) side of the wrist and not on the *radial* (thumb) side of the wrist where the wound image is depicted on the Shroud. Secondly, Barbet included a photograph of a cadaver that he had nailed to a cross in *Les cinq plaies du Christ*. If you examine a photo of the wrist area of this photograph, which I have provided, you will note that the nails are indeed nailed through the little finger side (*ulnar*) of the wrist and not on the thumb side (Figure 7-11). In addition, Barbet asked the master sculptor, Villandre, to

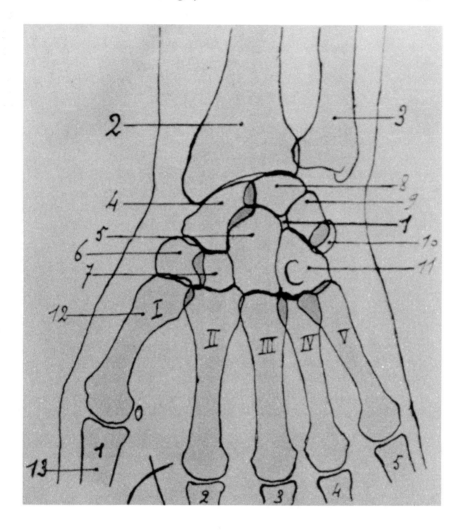

Figure 7-10

Diagram of wrist.

From Barbet's Le cinq plaies du Christ, *showing Destot's space. The anatomy labelled in the book: (1) espace libre mesocarpien de Destot (Destot's space). (2) radius. (3) cubitus. (4) scaphoide. (5) grand os. (6) trapeze. (7) trapezoid. (8) semi-lunare. (9) pyramidal. (10) pisiforme. (11) os crochu. (12) metacarpiens. (13) premiere phalanges.*

make a crucifix according to "precise information" he would give him. This was accomplished to Barbet's complete satisfaction. Note in Figure 7-12 that the nail again appears on the ulnar side of the wrist.

In support of the Destot space hypothesis, Barbet indicated that the soldiers were trained experts at crucifixion and alluded to the fact that they would know precisely where Destot's space was

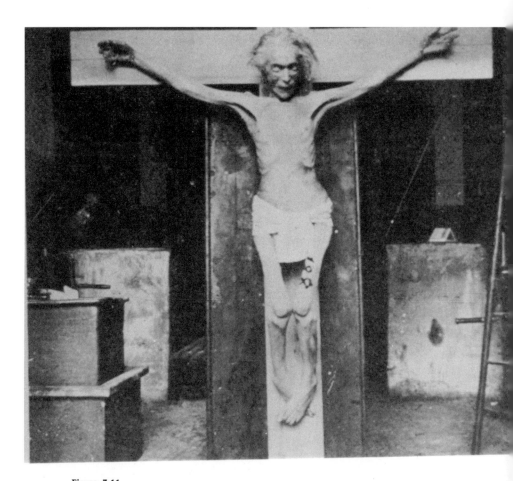

Figure 7-11
Cadaver suspended on cross by Barbet.
From Barbet's Le cinq plaies du Christ. *Note the nail is on the ulnar (little finger) side of the wrist and not the radial (thumb) side as depicted on the Shroud of Turin.*

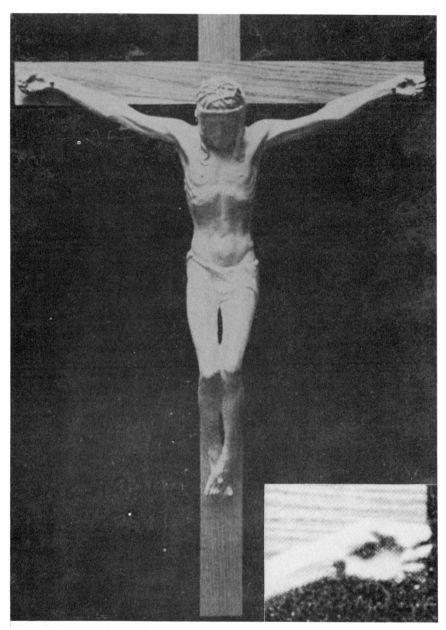

Figure 7-12

Villandre's crucifix.

From A Doctor at Calvary. *The cross was constructed from precise information given to Villandre by Barbet. Inset: Closeup of wrist showing site of entry of the nail. Again note the nail is on the ulnar (little finger) side of the wrist, not the radial side.*

located, suggesting that they would have used it routinely. This supposition is challenged by early historical accounts that indicate that crucifixion was done in many different ways* and also by the evidence that the crucified Jew, dating back to A.D. 7 in the Giv'at ha Mivtar excavation of the Jewish Quarter of Jerusalem by the Israel Exploration Society, was nailed between the radius and ulnar bones (see Figure 7-13). In developing the hypothesis that the nail passed through Destot's space, Barbet made his *second serious anatomical error*. He indicated that when he drove the nail through Destot's space, anywhere from one half to two thirds of the trunk of the *median nerve* was severed. If the nail passed through Destot's space, the trunk of the *median nerve would not* be severed because anatomically, the trunk of the median nerve runs along the wrist on the radial (thumb) side of the wrist and along the thenar furrow into the palm (Figures 7-3 and 7-4). To locate the *median nerve* on your own hand, bend your wrist forward and note that a cordlike structure, the palmaris longus tendon becomes very prominent. The median nerve is located on the radial (thumb) side of this ligament. If Barbet was not striking the median nerve, when he drove the square nails through the wrist, then what nerve was he cutting? The most likely nerve was a branch of the ulnar nerve that runs along the ulnar (little finger) side of the wrist since this nerve or a branch of it would most likely be in the area of Destot's space.

IF IT DID NOT GO THROUGH DESTOT'S SPACE, WHERE DID IT GO?

There are three possibilities that would be in accord with the scriptural point of view; the upper palm area, the wrist area, and the region between the radius and ulna. But would not the wrist area and the region between the radius and ulna be in contradiction to both the historical and scriptural accounts? In the ancient literature, Lipsius and other authors, painters and sculptors related that it was the hands that were transfixed in crucifixion, and the scriptures state that Jesus was nailed through his hands; "See my hands and my feet, that it is I myself" (Luke 24–39) and "He showed them his hands and side . . . "Then he said to Thomas, "Put your finger here, and see my hands. . ." (John 20:20–27)

---

*Seneca related "I see crosses there, not just one kind but made in many different ways; some have their victims with head down to the ground; some impale their private parts; others stretch out their arms on the gibbet."

"they pierced my hands and my feet" (Psalm 22:16). This presents no major obstacle because the word hand has always been defined anatomically as composite of the fingers, palm, dorsum (back of the hand) and wrist. Moreover, even the area between the radius and ulna would also be acceptable because the original translation of hand also included the front of the arm (Zorell's *Lexicon Hebraicum et Aramaicum* and Liddell-Scott's *Greek-English Lexicon*, 7th Edition, Harper Brothers, New York, 1883). The viability of this area was demonstrated when, as previously related, the excavation in the Jewish Quarter of the Old City of Jerusalem of a crucified man dating to A.D. 7 revealed evidence of nailing through the forearm between the radius and the ulna, where the radius bone displayed a scratch produced by frictional gliding and concomitant compression of the nail (Figure 7–13). This is an actual case in which the wrist area was used as a nailing site at the time of Christ. This area between the radius and ulna is unusually strong and is used routinely in slaughter houses to hang cattle, pigs and other animals.

The hand wound image on the Shroud, however, narrows the possibilities: through the radial (thumb) side of the wrist (not Destot's space), or through the upper part of the palm angled toward the wrist. Both of these areas are extremely strong, being capable of holding many hundreds of pounds. It is also of interest that both areas are in accord with the revelations of St. Brigit, "My son's hands were pierced at the spot where the bone was most solid."

RADIAL SIDE OF THE WRIST

In this instance, the nail could pass through the radial (thumb) side of the wrist through a space created by four other carpal bones; the *navicular, lunate, greater multangular* and *capitate bones,* emerging in the region of the hand wound image shown on the Shroud. This is a very strong area. The trunk of the median nerve would most likely be damaged by this path.

UPPER PART OF THE PALM

There are several reasons why the palm of the hand would be the most plausible region for the site of nailing in the case of Jesus Christ, since now it can be shown that the upper part of the palm would easily support the weight of the body on the cross. First of

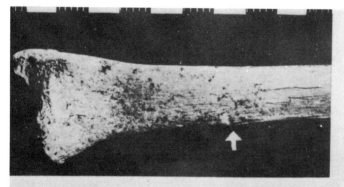

A : Distal end of the
bone, showing the scratch
duced by friction betwee
bone and the nail.

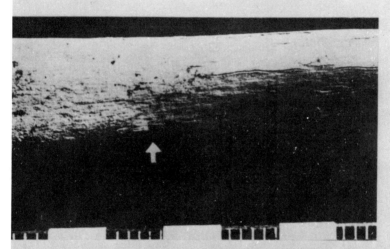

B : Detail of A

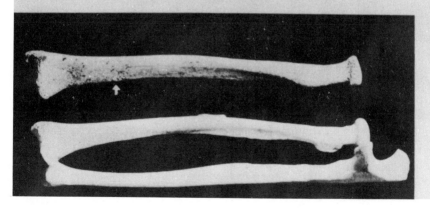

Figure 7-13
Radius bone (A and B).
Shows a friction scratch produced by a nail passing between the bone and nail
from the skeletal remains of a crucified man (A.D. 7) from Giv'at ha Mivtar.
(Courtesy of Israel Exploration Society.)

all, it is the location where most people through the centuries have perceived the wound to be, based on the Scriptures. Second, it is where artists depicted the nails in their artistic pieces (Figure 6-1). Third, it is where most of the stigmatists, like St. Francis of Assisi, Padre Pio, Theresa of Konnersruth, St. Catherine of Siena, Catherine of Ricci, Louise Lateau, etc., throughout the centuries have displayed their wounds. * Fourth, it assures that no bones are broken in accord with Exodus 12:46 and Numbers 9:12, and, last, it explains the apparent lengthening of the fingers of the Turin Shroud because of nail compression at this area.

Unfortunately, there is a great misunderstanding of the hand wound image on the Shroud. At the outset it must be firmly understood that the *hand wound image* is on the back of the hand and only depicts the exit of the nail, not its entrance (Figure 8-2). This tells us that *we do not specifically know where the entrance site is.* Therefore, even though the wound image is depicted on the wrist area, this *does not* preclude the palm area as the point of entry unless we are postulating that the nail passed vertically through the middle of the palm into the *patibulum* of the cross. *In this case, we would have to say no* because the nail would not be in the right place to create the hand image on the Shroud and the palms would not support the body on the cross according to the mathematical considerations discussed previously, to the observations of artists who found that the nails ripped through the hands of cadavers they nailed to crosses as models for their work, to anatomical considerations relating to the structure of the wrist, to the revelations of St. Brigit among other mystics, and to the experiments of Barbet on freshly amputated arms.

The upper part of the palm is, however, a different story because there is a path from the upper part of the palm to the exact site shown on the Shroud. Let us demonstrate this. If you open your hands, palms up, you will notice bulky prominences extending into the hand from the base of the thumbs. These masses are called the *thenar eminence muscles* (Figure 7-2), which cause the thumbs to *flex* (that is, bend into the palms). Now touch your thumb to the tip of

---

*It is noted that the only two stigmatists that are known to have their wounds in the wrist area include brother Gino Buresi of Rome and an unidentified American priest both of whom received their stigmata in recent years following the multitude of articles that quote Barbet's hypothesis that the nails pierced the wrists since the palms could not support the weight of the body.

your little finger and you will note a deep furrow at the base of the *thenar eminence muscles* called the *thenar furrow.* If a nail is driven into this furrow, a few centimeters from where the furrow begins at the wrist, with the point of the nail angled at ten to fifteen degrees toward the wrist and slightly toward the thumb (Figure 7-14, 7-15), there is a natural inclination of the nail to drive into an area created by the *metacarpal bone* of the index finger and the *capitate* and *lesser multangular* bones of the *carpus* (wrist), which we have coined the "Z" area (see Figure 7-16). The space is expanded as the nail passes through and exits at a point corresponding exactly to the hand wound image. I demonstrated this over thirty years ago in the

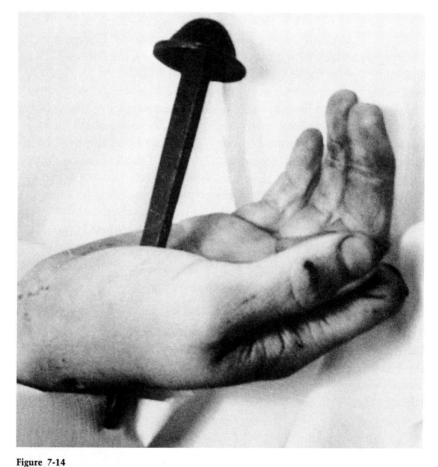

Figure 7-14
Nail through the palm, front.
A duplicate of an actual Roman nail passes through the thenar furrow at 10- to 15-degree angle inclined toward the wrist. This passes through the Z-area. (See text.)

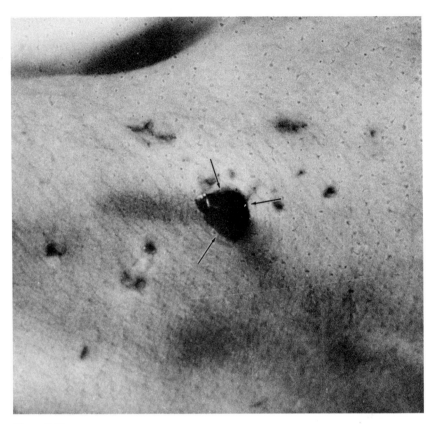

Figure 7-15
Nail through the palm, back.
Note that the nail driven through the thenar furrow in the previous photo exits at a point corresponding to the wound of the hand on the Turin Shroud.

anatomy dissection lab. Dissection of this area revealed that no bones were broken. A striking event confirmed this about two years ago in the medical examiner's office. A young lady had been brutally stabbed over her entire body. At autopsy, I found a defense wound on her hand where she had put her hand up to protect her face from the vicious onslaught. Examination of the hand wound revealed that she was stabbed in the thenar furrow in the palm of the hand. The knife passed through the "Z" area and the point of the knife exited at a site corresponding exactly to the hand image wound on the Shroud. X-rays of the area showed no broken bones. It is of interest to note that according to Barbet, Monsignor Alfonso Paleotto, Archbishop of Bologna, who accompanied St.

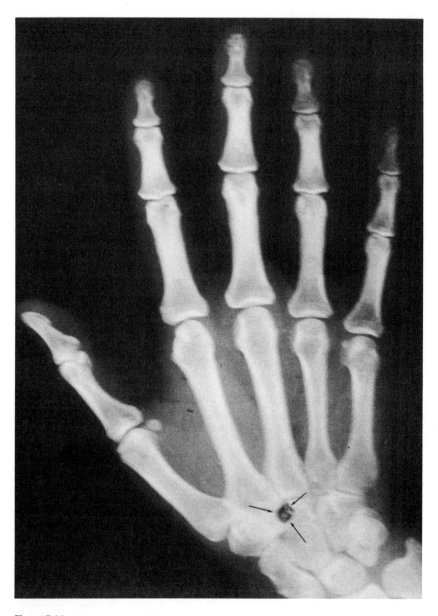

Figure 7-16

X-ray of the hand.

Note the site where the nail penetrated the palm of the hand at the thenar furrow and passed through the Z-area created by the two metatarsal bones (1 and 2) and the capitate and lesser multangular bones (3 and 4).

Charles Borromeo to Turin in 1598, also postulated that the nail would have entered the upper part of the palm obliquely, and pointing toward the arm it would have emerged where the Shroud depicts it. He published this in his book *Esplicatione del Sacro Lenzuolo Ove Fu Involto II Signore* in 1598. Barbet, however, severely criticized Paleotto's hypothesis as "anatomically impossible." This, of course, is absolute nonsense in view of my studies in the anatomical dissection lab and the unprecedented case from the medical examiner's office presented above.

THE EFFECTS OF NAILING THE PALMS

Clench the fist of your right hand tightly and bend the wrist forward. The palmaris longus tendon will jut out in the center of the front of the wrist in 90 percent of all individuals. This tendon is used anatomically to locate the median nerve, which lies just to the right of this tendon (see Figures 7-3 and 7-4). Note how this nerve runs from the wrist and fans out with a branch along the thenar furrow, as described previously. There is little doubt that branches of the median nerve would be injured causing a painfully disabling affliction called causalgia, which was classically described by Mitchell, Morehouse, and Keen in 1864 during the Civil War years. This syndrome was commonly seen during the war years after partial median nerve and other peripheral nerve injuries. The pain is described as a peculiar burning sensation that is so intense that even gentle contacts like clothing or air draft cause utter torture. The patient becomes completely preoccupied with avoiding any contact and holding the limb a particular way. This condition can completely destroy the morale of the most stoic of individuals. A study by Slesser revealed that the pain became more severe with increase in temperature and that none of his patients was able to tolerate direct sun rays. Profuse sweating of the palm also accompanies this syndrome. The only effective treatment has been found to be surgery to cut the sympathetic nerves. Prior to this treatment, numerous individuals became addicted to pain-killing drugs, and there were many cases of self-destruction.

HOW WOULD THE NAILING OF THE PALM AFFECT JESUS?

When the *exactor mortis* and his cronies (*quaternio*) nailed Jesus' hands to the *patibulum*, there was little doubt that branches of the median nerve were injured by the huge square iron nail that measured about fifteen centimeters in length. The pain would have been unrelenting and brutal with a severe burning sensation. All of the known inciting factors were present to aggravate the condition, including movements of air, the direct sun rays, the heat, the pressure of the nail constantly rubbing against the nerve, and the movements of the body on the cross. The pain would be markedly accentuated because of Jesus' utter fatigue. Monheim writes, "Of significant importance to the patient's pain threshold is fatigue. It has definitely been proved that patients who are rested and have had a good night's sleep previous to an unpleasant experience will have a much higher pain reaction threshold than an individual who is tired and worn." As you know, Jesus was up most of the night after his mental agony in the Garden of Olives, and this was followed by the brutal scourging, the crowning of thorns, and the trek to Calvary. Following these insults, he was in a severely exhausted condition with ubiquitous pains and in a state of trau-matic shock. It has often been repeated that if a person has pain in his head, kick him in the shin and he will forget about his head pain. The truth of the matter is that patients who are suffering multiple pains concomitantly have a magnification effect of their pain rather than an additive effect.

RAISING HIM ON THE CROSS

The method by which the crosspiece with the nailed victim was placed onto the upright is not clear, and no definitive refer-ences have been written in this regard. Various references in the historical literature to Latin phrases such as *ascendre crucem* (as-cend the cross) and the *patibulum suffixus* (fasten the *patibulum*) would indicate that the *exactor mortis* and his *quaternio* must have had some technique for executing this maneuver. Gorman indicates that two of the members of the team lifted each end of the *patibulum* and the third grasped Jesus by his waist to get him to his feet. He was then backed up to the *stipes* (upright) where two of the team lifted the crossbeam into a socket on the top of the *stipes* using forced sticks, while one of two individuals lifted Jesus around the body. Another possibility that was suggested is that a rope was tied around the body and the *patibulum* was hoisted onto the place over the *stipes* while two men helped by lifting the ends of this upright. This sounds impractical to me. It seems that there must have been an easier way, because when individuals are placed in a job that they are performing routinely, they soon find an easy way of doing it. I am sure they must have had a stairlike contraption of some sort, whereupon they made the one to be crucified climb up the stairs backward, while two members of the *quaternio* lifted the crosspiece and the third helped him up to the top step, whereupon the *patibulum* was set in place on the mortise. The steps could then be pulled away while the legs were held by the men. When a *sedile* was used, the task would have been easier, as he could straddle this while the *patibulum* was set in place and the feet nailed. This was not done in the case of Christ because the Passover and Sabbath were at hand and no procedure would have been used to prolong life. There are no reliable references about the practice of raising the entire cross; many references indicate that the *stipes* of *staticulum* were already in place, and some indicate that they were present in large numbers.

NAILING THE FEET

The main question is whether Jesus' feet were nailed separately using two nails or whether one foot was crossed on top of the other using a single nail, not whether his feet were nailed per se. None of the Gospels specifically relate that the feet were fastened with nails, but according to the revelations of St. Brigit, Jesus' feet were fixed with two nails.

It should be stressed at the outset that from a medical point of view it hardly seems important because the effects of each method would be similar. An evaluation of artistic pieces and other representations up to the twelfth century show the feet were nailed side by side in most, and Gregory of Tours in the sixth century writes of "Four Nails." Other early writers, including St. Gregory Nazianzen, St. Bonaventure and St. Anselme, however, support the three-nail theory, and many recent scientists, physicians, and authors who have studied the Turin Shroud favor the idea that one foot was placed on top of the other because of the odd inward position of the impression of the right foot at the tip and the left foot slightly shorter on the Turin Shroud. Gambesia, however, embraces a somewhat unusual two nail theory that holds that one nail pierced the metatarsal area of one foot with a second nail passing through the front of the ankle and passing through the heel. The fact of the matter is that the Romans had no single technique or uniform method in crucifixion, as previously indi-cated. The skeletal remains of the crucified man, which date back to about A.D. 7, bear this out vividly. According to Haas, both calcanei (heel) bones were pierced by a single nail (Figures 7-17–7-19). A restoration of the manner in which this individual was crucified is illustrated in Figures 7-20 and 7-21. Zias and Sekeles reappraised the studies of Haas using x-rays and found that the nail only passed through one heel bone. These reconstructions indicate that the victim straddled the upright with each foot nailed laterally to the cross (Figure 7-21). There have also been reports of crucified victims being nailed through the Achilles tendons, the large, strong tendons located at the back of the feet.

It would appear more logical that two nails were used to nail the feet of Jesus because it would have been easier to accomplish the task. Try the following maneuver. Lie flat on the floor and bend your knees. Note that the soles of your feet are now flush to the floor. Now, have someone hold your feet down and try to pull them away. You will note how difficult a task it is to free them, although your knees would be in full motion. Bend your knees and place one

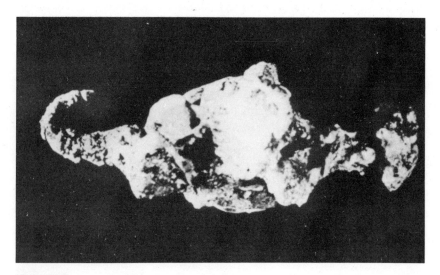

Figure 7-17
The heel (calcanean) bone of a crucified man
As discovered at the Giv'at ha Mivtar excavation. Notice the coating of thick calcareous crust.
(Courtesy of Israel Exploration Society and Mrs. Nicu Haas).

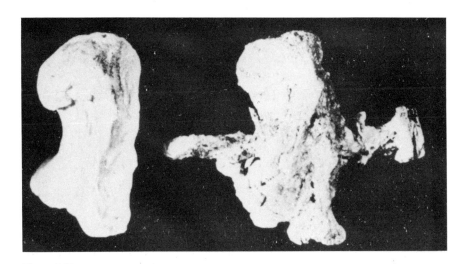

Figure 7-18
The heel (calcanean) bone of a crucified man.
After a first attempt of reconstruction, in comparison with an actual left calcanean bone.
(Courtesy of Israel Exploration Society and Mrs. Nicu Haas).

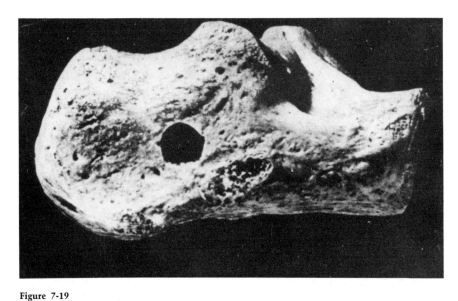

Figure 7-19
Heel bone showing perforation.
Actual left heel of the crucified victim of Giv'at ha Mivtar excavation showing the place of perforation at the side of the heel.
(Courtesy of Israel Exploration Society and Mrs. Nicu Haas).

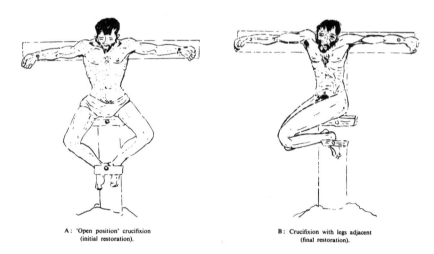

A : 'Open position' crucifixion
(initial restoration).

B : Crucifixion with legs adjacent
(final restoration).

Figure 7-20

Reconstructions of an A.D. 7 crucified man.

Reconstructions (initial and final) of the position on the cross established from the Giv'at ha Mivtar excavations.
(Courtesy of Israel Exploration Society and Mrs. Nicu Haas).

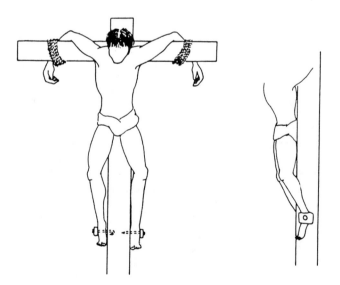

Figure 7-21

Reconstruction of A.D. 7 crucified man.
(Courtesy of Drs. Zia and Sekeles).

foot on top of the other and have someone hold your feet down. Now it becomes very difficult for your assistant to hold your feet. If you apply the same reasoning to crucifixion, you will find that after the hands are secured, the executioner would then merely bend the knees and, perhaps, initially tie the feet to the upright. It would be relatively easy to nail the feet with the direct back support of the upright and to allow the nails to be driven through the foot without breaking any bones. On the other hand, it would be extremely difficult, if the human being struggled, to hold one foot on top of the other and drive a nail through both feet, particularly without breaking any bones, because the alignment of both feet would have to be perfect. "They have pierced my hands and feet, I can count all my bones" (Psalms 22:16–17). (Please refer to Chapter 12 for an interpretive evaluation of the foot images.)

In our experiments on the cross, we have demonstrated how easily the feet become flush to the upright with strapping (Figure 7-22). It was also apparent during these studies that the feet felt almost glued to the cross in this position. There is support for this concept in the Syrian *Codex* of Rabula (A.D. 586), where the feet appear to be directly nailed to the *stipes*. The insistence by many authors that a *suppadenum* or foot support was necessary derives from their conclusions that Christ needed this device as a support to raise his body in order to breathe to prevent asphyxiation. Our experiments, however, detailed in the section on cause of death, demonstrated that merely strapping the soles of the feet flush to the *stipes* will support the body firmly without need for a *suppadenum* or foot support, proving that the *suppadenum* was unnecessary. The right foot image on the Turin Shroud is also contrary to the use of a *suppadenum*, otherwise, the whole sole could not have been flush to the Shroud. These experiments should serve to correct the misconception that a *suppadenum* was necessary.

THE EFFECTS OF SECURING THE FEET

In our experiments with individuals hanging on the cross, they felt marked cramping of the calf and thigh muscles with numbness of the feet after a short period of time hanging. Twitching was commonly noted, and after ten minutes the limbs felt cool. Straightening movements relieved the pain temporarily (refer to Chapter 19).

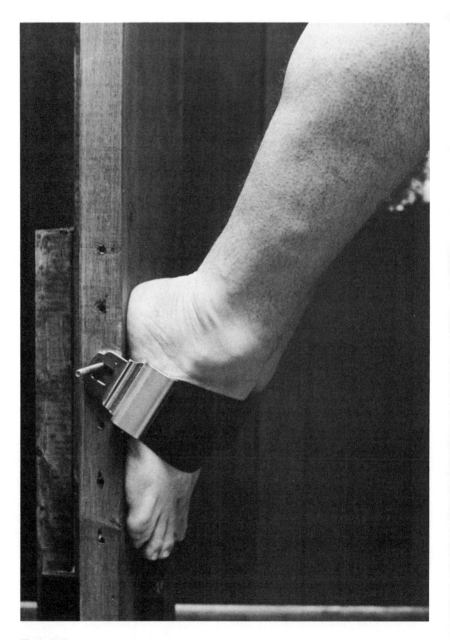

Figure 7-22
Position of feet during crucifixion.
Note that the soles are flush to the stipes (upright) by slight bending of the knees.

Some of the effects of nailing the feet may be somewhat similar to those of the hands discussed previously if any of the branches of the plantar nerves were injured. These nerves bifurcate down the foot with a branch on both sides of each metatarsal bone, and even slight injury would result in a causalgia syndrome, as described under the section on nailing the hand.

HOW WOULD THE NAILING OF THE FEET AFFECT JESUS?

The pain in Jesus' feet would have been severe with the iron nail pressing against the plantar nerves like "red hot pokers," similar to that suffered by the median nerve injuries during nailing of the hands. Even a slight movement would incite the incessant, burning pains. After a short period of time on the cross, the severe cramps, the numbness, and the coldness in the calves and thighs, caused by the compression by the bent knees, would force him to push up occasionally and attempt to straighten his legs. This would continue periodically throughout the entire period that Jesus was on the cross.

In conclusion, the Romans secured the hands by various modes during crucifixion—by the palms, the wrist, and the fore-arm. There is, however, little question that *Jesus was affixed to the cross through the palms of the hands* with the nails passing through the thenar furrow or groove and the point of the nail angles ten to fifteen degrees toward the wrist and slightly toward the thumb. This is a very sturdy region, as Christians have always perceived it to be, where it has always been displayed on the hands of stigmatists, where no bones are broken, and where the nail emerges at a point corresponding to the image on the Turin Shroud.

It is logical to assume that *both feet were nailed* separately and flush to the cross without being placed one on top the other because to do this is easier to execute, no bones are broken, and it would correspond to the earliest Christian references.

The pain suffered during transfixing of the palms and feet derives from the injury to the median nerves of the hands and the plantar nerves of the feet causing a disabling condition called causalgia, characterized by a brutal, burning, unrelenting pain that is aggravated by every movement on the cross, reducing the *cruciarius* to a wretched state.

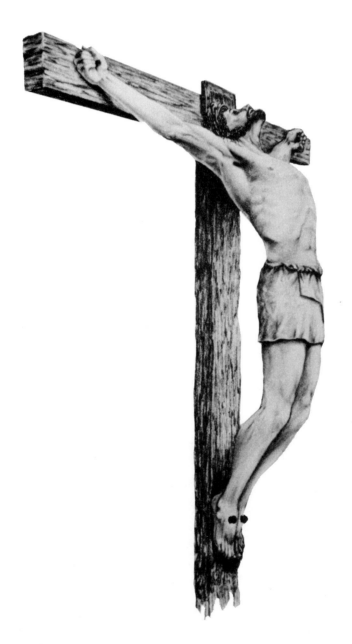

Figure 8-1
Arched position of crucifixion.
Drawing by Bruce Drummond.

8

Christ Is Crucified

The effects of hanging upon the cross are relatively complex, but if we carefully analyze the various concepts, theories, speculations, and experimental studies, we will gain a reasonably thorough idea of the suffering Christ experienced on the cross.

THE ASPHYXIATION (SUFFOCATION) THEORY

The most widely held theory that has been propagated as the cause of death is the *asphyxiation theory,* also referred to as the suffocation theory. This concept indicates that the position on the cross is incompatible with breathing because the air would be trapped in the lung following inspiration (breathing in), thereby requiring the victim to raise his body in order to breathe. This act of raising and lowering would continue until exhaustion set in and death would occur because of asphyxiation (suffocation). The unfortunate part of this concept is that it is based on a priori rather than a posteriori reasoning and has been found to be completely untenable when tested empirically. Father Weyland, the famous sculptor who performed a series of suspensions on the cross, with himself and several volunteers as subjects, in order to gain true perspective for his artistic pieces, aptly stated, "Conjectures and theories not backed up by realistic experiments always left me cold."

This state of affairs perhaps derives from the paucity of scien-tific studies regarding the medical aspects of Shroud of Turin research and the failure of valid experimental studies that might challenge the validity of proposed theories. Many scientists fre-quently forget that it is their duty whenever possible to provide experimental support for their hypotheses.

Asphyxiation is a physiological and chemical state that results from an inability of a living organism to obtain adequate oxygen for cell metabolism and to eliminate excess carbon dioxide. Usually, a six to ten minute span of complete respiratory obstruction causes irreversible brain damage and perhaps death.

The asphyxiation or suffocation theory was first propounded by LeBec in 1925. He theorized that the position on the cross with the arms overhead would immobilize the chest making it difficult to breathe out, thereby suffocating the person. This was supported by Hynek in 1936. It was, however, Barbet who refined the theory and gave it its greatest impetus by presenting it in a very simple and attractive way. It was based on three major a priori factors he claimed confirmed this hypothesis: a.) *Austro-German army* and *Dachau concentration camp hangings*; b.) the *bifurcation pattern* corresponding to the hand wound image on the Shroud; and c.) *the crurifragium (skelekopia)*, breaking of the legs.

AUSTRO-GERMAN ARMY AND DACHAU CONCENTRATION CAMP HANGINGS

Hynek attempted to confirm LeBec's contentions by an obser-vation he made during World War I when he served in the Austro-German army. Punishment was doled out to soldiers by hanging the condemned by his wrists with his feet barely raised off the ground. After a short time, violent contractions of all of the muscles occurred causing severe muscle spasms. The tortured individual had extreme difficulty breathing out, causing asphyxiation. This lasted for about ten minutes at which time he was usually cut down. Barbet reinforced Hynek's observations with the testimony of two prisoners from the Dachau concentration camp who indicated that the condemned man was hung by his hands with his feet some distance from the ground, which caused difficulty breathing out and required him to raise himself by his hands in order to expire (breathe out). He would raise and drop his body continuously until he became exhausted and succumbed to asphyxiation.

Both observations are very interesting but would only be valid when applied to an individual whose arms were suspended directly above his head. Moreover, *they in no way support the asphyxiation hypothesis.* Applying these observations to the asphyxiation theory is like comparing apples to oranges. In one instance the hands and arms are raised above the head to support the weight of the body. This is an entirely different situation than that of a person suspended at an angle of sixty to seventy degrees with the *stipes* (upright). If a body is suspended by the hands-raised-above-the-head position, there unquestionably is breathing difficulty. Therefore, if it were determined that Jesus' arms were suspended directly above his head then I would have no difficulty accepting the asphyxiation hypothesis as the probable cause of death. Barbet, however, based his hypothesis on an angle of sixty-five degrees with the *stipes.* This is also confirmed by the photograph of the cadaver that Barbet nailed to the cross (Figure 7-11) and by Villandre's crucifix (Figure 7-12).

An attempt to confirm the asphyxiation theory was made by Moedder, an Austrian radiologist from Cologne who suspended medical students by the wrists. With their hands above their heads, less than forty inches apart on a horizontal bar using cloth bands, the students became pale within a few minutes and the vital capacity of the lungs decreased from 5.2 to 1.5 liters with shallow respirations, and there was a decrease in blood pressure and a rising pulse rate. If the students could rest for a few minutes alternating with three minutes of hanging they could last longer. Moedder concluded that orthostatic collapse occurs within six minutes if the students were not allowed to stand. Again this experiment has no relation to crucifixion since the hands were suspended above the head and not at the crucifixion angle of sixty-five to seventy degrees. The results of Moedder's experiments merely confirmed that asphyxiation would occur if the *cruciarius* was suspended by his hands above his head.

BIFURCATION PATTERN

The bifurcation pattern on the hand wound image of the Shroud (Figure 8-2) was interpreted by Barbet as representing two positions that Jesus assumed in order to breathe while he was on the cross. He postulated that Jesus was unable to expire (breathe out), as was observed at Dachau, because the air was trapped in inspira-

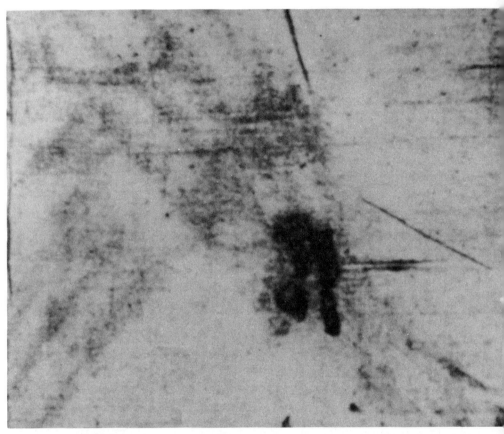

Figure 8-2
Shroud of Turin, hand wound image.
This is an enlargement of the back of the hand, therefore, it does not represent the entrance *wound made by the nail but the* exit *wound (see text). Note the bifurcation pattern of the blood image.*

tion (breathing in). He therefore had to push up with his feet in order to expel the air from his lungs. The interpretation of the bifurcation pattern is utterly ridiculous because *this pattern is located on the back of the hand—not on the front.* Why should that matter? Very simply, the back of the hand is pressed against the *patibulum* of the cross by the nailing. How in the world can you get a double flow of blood? The heart is beating and is constantly extruding blood through the wound and I assure the reader that the hand is heavily endowed with blood vessels in vast networks constantly feeding from major blood vessels on both sides of the hand. This would create a large blood smudge. Contrary to Barbet's statement that the effusion of blood would be moderate and entirely venous because the nail would hit no important artery, there are important arteries present. This is supported by British Home Office Pathologist James Cameron, a forensic pathologist who indicated that a nail passing through the area of the median nerve would most likely hit a main artery.

The nail itself would afford a degree of hemostasis (control of bleeding) by exerting pressure within the wound but every movement on the cross would result in episodes of oozing and over several hours there would be a substantial blood collection. Even tiny wounds bleed profusely during heart activity. We see this on a daily basis in the medical examiner's office. One recent case is exemplary. A young lady who slightly nicked a superficial vein in her neck with a small wood-carving knife went to bed apparently in the belief that she would bleed to death. She bled so profusely that her face, neck, hair, and chest and the bed linen were saturated with blood.

Another important point that militates against the two positions causing a "double flow of blood" is the fact that the wrist does not change its angle on the cross even if the victim had to raise himself in order to breathe. The reason—*the arms bend at the elbows and not at the wrists.* We confirmed this during our suspension experiments even though the hands were not firmly bound to the *patibulum* as they were during the crucifixion when the *cruciarius* was nailed with a square nail, which was forced between the bones and ligaments of the hand and nailed solidly into the cross (see suspension experiments below).

An additional consideration derives from the excruciating pain that would have been experienced if the *cruciarius* attempted to raise himself by putting an amount of pressure equal to the weight of the body against the nails in the feet. This pain would have been brutal.

The reason for this bifurcation effect became obvious during observations in the medical examiner's office. When clots within bullet wounds, stab wounds, and auto accident injuries of this area of the wrist are disturbed, rivulets of blood are noted to run from the wounds. In one case I investigated several years ago, I placed a metal probe into a wrist wound, disturbing a clot made by a bullet. The body was carried down the stairs and removed to the morgue. When I saw the body of the deceased the next day, there was a bifurcated flow of blood from the wound to both sides of the ulnar styloid protuberance (the bump on the little finger side of the back of the wrist). Thus, I suggest that when the nail was removed from Jesus' wrist, a clot or smudge of dried blood was disturbed, causing an oozing and divergence of the blood to flow to the ulnar styloid protuberance.

BREAKING OF THE LEGS

The breaking of the legs called *skelokopia* or *crurifragium* was Barbet's final a priori argument to support his theory that Jesus died of asphyxiation. According to Barbet, if the legs were broken, then the *cruciarius* would be unable to raise himself to breathe. This is certainly an attractive thesis considering the fact that the Romans broke the legs of the two thieves who were crucified on both sides of Jesus, who was spared this because he was already dead: ". . . but when they came to Jesus and saw that he was already dead, they did not break his legs." (John 19:33).

The *crurifragium* was strikingly demonstrated on the skeletal remains of the A.D. 7 crucified man (see Figure 8-3). There is evidence that the legs were not broken to prevent the victim from raising himself in order to breathe. If you carefully examine the final restoration of Haas (Figure 7-20) or Zias and Sekeles (Figure 7-21), you will note that the body was already in a maximally lifted position. Zias and Sekeles, however, claim that Haas' interpretation that the broken bones are indicative of the *crurifragium* is incorrect since the breaks are situated at different angles, indicating that they must have occurred after death. This interpretation is, however, untenable since this pattern indicates that the victim received more than one blow at different angles. The ritual of *crurifragium* was usually performed at a time when the victim was near death. This would be the *coup de grace* blow that would hasten death by causing severe traumatic shock, and in some instances, a fatty embolism in a person near death. Since the *cruciarius* is in a severely weakened condition of shock, the breaking of the legs would deepen the level of traumatic shock with a consequent drop in blood pressure and rapid development of congestion in the lower extremities resulting in unconsciousness, coma, and death. Historically, *skelokopia* is believed to have been performed after all crucifixions including those with a *sedile* (saddle) who had been suspended for long periods of time. Surely, breaking the legs of

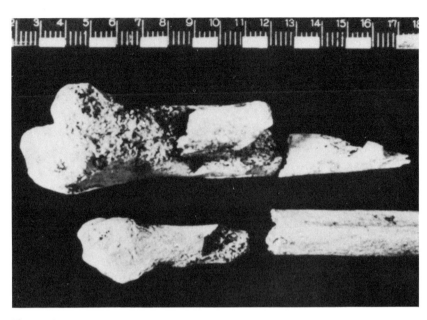

Figure 8-3
Crurifragium of tibia and fibula bones.
Breaking of the legs (crurifragium or skelokopia) of the crucified man from the Giv'at ha Mivtar Excavation.
(Courtesy of Israel Society and Mrs. Nicu Haas).

victims on a *sedile* would be contradictory if the purpose of breaking the legs was to prevent them from raising themselves with their legs in order to breathe. The *crurifragium* was a "finishing off" procedure for both the victim still on the cross or following removal from the cross. Some authors believe that the *crurifragium* was done to prevent the victim from crawling away following removal from the cross so that wild animals could devour them and others indicate that it was also used as a form of punishment.

CONCLUSION

Huxley once made reference to *"the slaying of a beautiful hypothesis by an ugly fact."** The asphyxiation theory is a prime example of this.

*Collected Essays, vol. 8, *Discourses, Biological and Geological,* Macmillan, London, 1894.

9

Experiments on the Cross

If the asphyxiation theory is untenable, then what would be the effects of suspension on the cross? To answer these questions, a series of experiments were designed using human volunteers between the ages of twenty and thirty-five.

THE CROSS

It was necessary to perform our experiments on a cross that would allow close correspondence to the position of crucifixion by providing the appropriate angle of the arms with the upright, afford a means of securing the hands to the *patibulum* without constricting the wrists, and enable the feet to be appropriately secured to the upright. A sturdy cross, with the *stipes* ninety-two inches high and a *patibulum* seventy-eight inches wide with the base secured with reinforced angle iron was built for me by the late Father Peter Weyland, S.V.D., noted sculptor and sindologist. The *patibulum* contained a series of small numbered holes at close intervals to allow for different arm spans, because the appropriate angle depends on individual variations of shoulder and arm structure. Each hole was drilled on a slightly downward angle, from front to back, enabling long bolts to be inserted in the appropriate holes from back to front. In this way bolts could be inserted from back to front in an upward direction to avoid slippage by leather gauntlets.

THE GAUNTLETS

Special leather gauntlets were used for suspension to eliminate the need for gripping with the hands. These cuffs could be laced around a gloved hand without compromising the blood supply to this area and provided a hole between the base of the fingers that could be placed over each bolt on the *patibulum* (see Figure 9-1).

SECURING THE FEET

A series of closely spaced holes were drilled along the sides of the *patibulum* over a two-foot range in the foot region so that a special belt could be placed at different levels to secure the feet firmly against the upright.

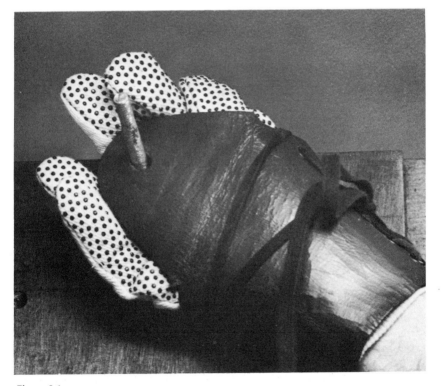

Figure 9-1
Closeup of hand gauntlet.
This is used to hold the volunteer on the cross. (See text.)

EXPERIMENTAL DESIGN

A series of critical experiments were designed to obtain the following information:

(1) the exact angle of the arms with the upright of the cross underneath,

(2) visual observations of the various positions assumed on the cross from the beginning to the end of the suspension,

    (a) evidence of the presence of muscle twitchings and muscle contractions, the parts of the body involved, and the time of appearance of these twitchings and contractions.

    (b) observations of the chest (thorax) and diaphragm for the type of breathing, chest movements, difficulty breathing, and so forth,

    (c) color of the face for evidence of oxygenation or lack of oxygenation to the head region,

    (d) the presence of sweating,

(3) subjective complaints including pain location, psychological feelings, breathing difficulties,

(4) respiratory evaluation,

    (a) auscultation (stethoscope examination) of the lungs to determine the presence of lung pathology,

    (b) determination of the percent oxygen saturation of the blood at rest and during the entire suspension procedure to determine empirically if adequate oxygenation is present with time during suspension using a special instrument called an ear oximeter,

    (c) determination of the respiratory quotient, which is the volume of carbon dioxide eliminated by the body during a given time divided by the volume of oxygen that is absorbed, by collecting the expired air in a large bag called a Douglas bag and subsequently analyzing the air (the amount of carbon dioxide and oxygen in the air expired and the total air intake).

    (d) determination of lung ventilation and the vital capacity, which is the maximum volume of air that can be expelled from the lungs after full inspiration (breathing in),

    (e) measuring the blood lactic acid level before and during suspension as an indication of muscle activity due to oxygen lack and carbon dioxide production,

(5) determination of the cardiovascular effects, which include,

(a) auscultation of the heart (examination with a stethoscope) to determine any abnormalities of rhythm, presence of murmurs, gallops, or other abnormal sounds,

(b) blood pressure determinations using an electronic sphygmomanometer (blood pressure unit) with double transducers (for increased sensitivity) before and throughout the hanging procedure to determine if there is a progressive rise, fall, plateau, and so forth of the blood pressure,

(c) monitoring the cardiac (heart) activity with a monitor containing a digital display of the electrocardiogram pattern, display of the pulse rate, and automatic half-minute printouts of the EKG strips, and

(6) blood chemistries including certain enzymes contained in the muscle, heart, liver, and other organs as an additional determination of the skeletal muscle activity, presence of cardiac damage, and so forth. These enzymes include: Creatinine phosphokinase (CPK) and isoenzymes of CPK (skeletal muscle and heart muscle enzymes), lactic dehydrogenase, serum glutamic oxaloacetic transaminase, and serum glutamic pyruvic transaminase (enzymes present in heart, liver and other areas of the body).

Human volunteers between the ages of twenty and thirty-five were given a physical examination and resting values were obtained which included, a twelve lead electrocardiogram, pulse rate, blood pressure, stethoscope examination (with capacity and ear oximetry values), arterial blood gases, and venous blood chemistries.

PREPARATION OF THE VOLUNTEERS

Areas of the chest were shaved, the skin prepared, and special heart electrodes were glued to the chest and attached to a stress-testing instrument that monitored the electrocardiogram patterns and heart rate both at rest and during hanging and provided electrocardiogram strips automatically every minute (Figure 9-2). A blood pressure cuff containing double transducers was wrapped around the upper arm, and the cables were attached to an electronic blood pressure unit for obtaining the resting blood pressure and blood pressure throughout the hanging process. Attached to each ear was an ear oximeter probe (Figure 9-3), which gave the blood oxygen level at all times prior to hanging and all during the

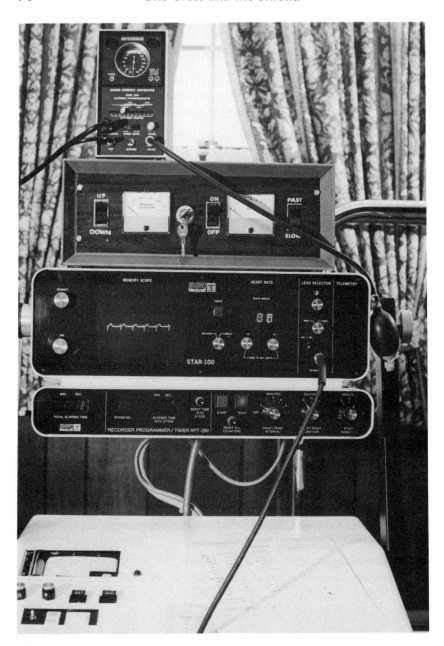

Figure 9-2

Cardiac monitor and electronic blood pressure recorder.
There is a monitoring screen on electrocardiogram (EKG) display. Heart rate (88).
The rectangular unit at the top is the blood pressure unit. The white unit at the
bottom of the picture is an automatic electrocardiogram recorder that records an
EKG strip automatically every half minute.

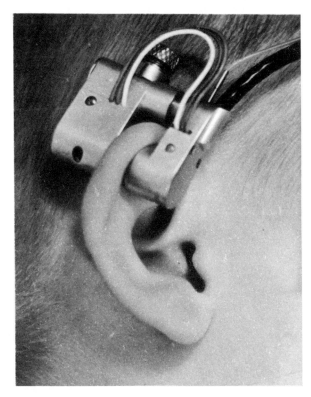

Figure 9-3
Ear oximeter.
This is used throughout the suspensions to record the oxygen saturation in the blood.
(Courtesy of the Waters Corporation).

suspension process. The gauntlets, as described above, were placed over gloves and laced securely (Figure 7-12).

Each volunteer was instructed to inform us of any breathing difficulties, pains of any kind, muscle cramps, or any other problems. They were also requested not to attempt to lift the body up at any time by straightening their legs.

MANNING THE CROSS

The volunteer climbed up on a high stool or table, and his arms were outstretched against the *patibulum* to find the numbered hole corresponding to his arm length. The bolts were then inserted into these holes and the holes of the gauntlets were placed over the bolts. The stool or table was gently removed and the body was allowed to suspend fully. The knees were then bent by sliding the heels upward against the *stipes* until the soles were flush to the cross at the lowest point possible and the feet were strapped at this point with the seat belts (Figure 9-4).

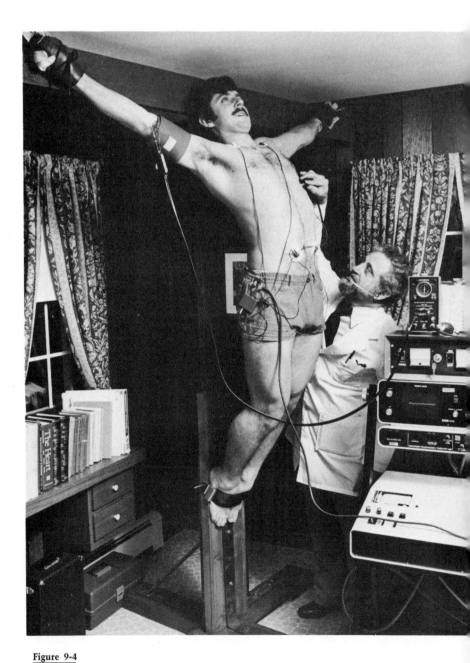

Figure 9-4
Experimental suspension on the cross.
Note the arched position, with the head back, assumed by the volunteer to relieve the pull on the shoulders. The back never touches the cross.

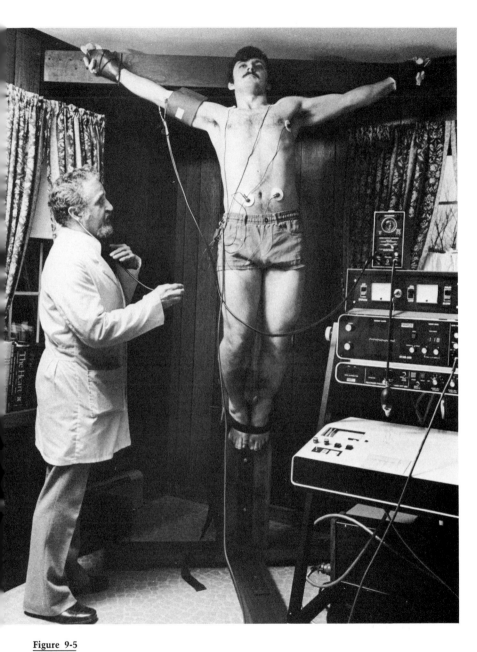

Figure 9-5

Experimental suspension on the cross.
Constant monitoring is performed throughout the suspension.

An emergency crash cart complete with defibrillator, cardiac medications, and intubation equipment was on hand to provide for the volunteer's safety. Individuals were stationed to the right and left of the volunteer in case of an emergency.

METHODS AND RESULTS

ANGLE OF SUSPENSION

Photographs were taken of the volunteers, and the exact angles created by the arms with the vertical (*stipes* or *staticulum*) of the cross were measured on the photographs. There was an individual variation of the angle ranging from sixty to seventy degrees. Therefore, the amount of pull on each arm would range from 175 to 256 pounds in an individual weighing 175 pounds (Table 7-1 in Chapter 7).

An additional experiment was performed on several of the volunteers. They were told to push themselves up with their feet, as indicated in Barbet's asphyxiation theory, in order to observe the angle of the wrist in both positions.

VISUAL OBSERVATIONS

A striking observation noted in all of the suspended volunteers was that the body did not touch the cross except in the shoulder region where there was very slight contact (see Figure 9-4). A fascinating pose that was periodically assumed was an arched configuration, with the top of the head arched backward against the upright, so that the top of the head actually touched the *stipes*. This reason for assuming this position was to relieve the severe strain on the shoulder region. As far as I can ascertain, this arched position has never been reported previously, and it was so striking that I decided to have a crucifix carved and drawings made (see Figure 8-1).

Throughout the suspension, the volunteers were constantly shifting their bodies and assuming various positions to relieve the strain and cramps from the shoulders, arms, legs, and knees. Muscle twitchings were commonly noted in the upper arms, the chest muscles and thighs of most volunteers, particularly after seven to eight minutes. In some cases, there was a complaint of "pins and needles" in the hands, arms, and in some of the areas that were twitching.

The chest appeared fixed, and abdominal (diaphragmatic) breathing became very obvious. There was an increase in the breathing rate, which became noticeable after four minutes, gradually increased in intensity to about four to five times normal and appeared to taper off at three to four times normal after seven to eight minutes.

The face appeared somewhat flushed after five to seven minutes, indicative of sufficient blood circulation to the head region. There was no evidence of cyanosis (blue coloration of the lips and fingernails), and the individual appeared in no respiratory distress.

Between six and eight minutes after the beginning of suspension, a marked sweating reaction became manifest in most individuals, which encompassed the entire body and in some instances actually drenched the volunteers, running off the toes to form a puddle on the floor. This occurred even though the experiments were conducted in an air-conditioned room (70° Fahrenheit).

SUBJECTIVE COMPLAINTS

Each volunteer was requested to submit the subjective complaints that he experienced during the suspension procedure, to include feelings of pain, location of pains, psychological feelings, breathing difficulties, and so forth. The most common complaint was the severe pull on the shoulders and pain in the knees, feet, and wrists. All of the subjects were aware of their breathing and indicated that their chests felt rigid, breathing was abdominal, and their inspirations appeared short with longer expirations. There were no feelings of any breathing difficulty even after forty minutes of suspension. Sometimes jerky respirations were felt in the diaphragmatic area during the first few minutes of suspension, which calmed down shortly thereafter. In every instance when the volunteer felt there might be a breathing difficulty, this was always at the beginning of the procedure and disappeared later during suspension or did not appear at all during subsequent hangings. This was commonly accepted by the volunteers as a psychological reaction due to fear in the early part of the hanging procedure that disappeared later in the hanging procedure and in subsequent suspensions. Some individuals indicated that the hanging procedure was extremely nerve-racking, and some experienced a feeling of panic.

The pain varied from person to person depending on their own physical development. There was aching and numbness throughout the body, and a few individuals felt as if their shoulders were being pulled out of their sockets. Other individuals experienced more pain in the lower part of their arms, others in the biceps, triceps, and deltoid muscles of the arm and shoulder. It was very interesting that in many individuals, the arms felt very tight at the beginning of the procedure, but flabby and flaccid after several minutes. Some of the individuals complained of extreme pain in the elbows and ankles and of forearm numbness, but the latter disappeared later in the suspension. Most of the volunteers indicated that their legs felt cold below the knee after twelve to fifteen minutes and took several minutes to warm after getting down.

EFFECTS ON THE RESPIRATORY SYSTEM

AUSCULTATION

The lungs were clear to auscultation (listening with stethoscope), and there was no evidence of any pathological sounds during the entire suspension procedure.

PERCENTAGE OF OXYGEN SATURATION IN THE BLOOD

The oxygen saturation of the blood is an important test that determines if the individual suspended on the cross is obtaining an adequate amount of oxygen. If the oxygen saturation begins to diminish significantly with time on the cross, this would confirm that the individual is obtaining insufficient oxygenation to the lungs and would add support to the asphyxiation theory. On the other hand, if it remains constant or increases, the converse would be true. The amount of oxygen in the blood was determined throughout the suspension using an instrument called an ear oximeter (Figure 9-3), which measures the light absorption of the hemoglobin (the oxygen-carrying component in a red blood corpuscle) at two different light frequencies and affords a direct value of the percent of oxygen saturation in the arteries of the blood at all times. The ear probe is clamped to the ear of the individual on the cross, as indicated in the diagram, and a light bulb heats the ears, dilating the arterioles (tiny arteries), so that the flow of blood is so rapid that very little deoxygenation occurs in the capillaries.

The results of this study revealed an increasing oxygen saturation in every case. An example of the findings in a typical hanging revealed that the control saturation level (reading prior to hanging) was 97 percent and rose to 99.5 percent in fifteen minutes during suspension. This was fully explained by the fact that the individuals progressively hyperventilated during this time to an average of three to four times normal after about eight minutes of suspension.

RESPIRATORY QUOTIENT (R.Q.)

The respiratory quotient is the ratio of the volume of carbon dioxide evolved from the lungs divided by the volume of oxygen absorbed from the lungs in one minute and reflects an excess in metabolism during the period of exertion. The oxygen consumption, the carbon dioxide output, and the total air volume breathed were determined both at rest and after twelve minutes of exercise by having the individuals breathe into a Douglas bag, which collects the gases and allows their measurement. The results of this experiment revealed a significant increase, consistent with marked muscular activity. Large amounts of carbon dioxide are released from the lungs because of the increased lactic acid levels caused by increased muscular activity with an oxygen deficit to the muscles.

RESPIRATORY AND VENTILATORY ACTIVITY

The lung ventilation (breathing) increases proportionately to the degree of muscular activity, rises in body temperature, fall in oxygen level, increase in carbon dioxide, increase in lactic acid, reflexes from many of the joints, and impulses from the higher brain centers produced by emotional factors. The volunteers showed an increased hyperventilation during the first six minutes, which reached a steady state of about four to five times normal at about eight minutes. The vital capacity (maximum volume of air that can be expelled from the lungs after full inspiration) showed a slight decrease after two to four minutes and remained constant thereafter.

LACTIC ACID CONTENT

The lactic acid of the blood increased progressively to about three and a half times normal after fifteen minutes of hanging. This is an indication of the marked muscular activity due to a lack of oxygen to the muscles. The initial rise of lactic acid is a powerful respiratory stimulant that causes hyperventilation in order to increase the oxygen supply. One must realize, however, that the increase in lactic acid level does not necessarily mean that the blood oxygen level is low because even under conditions of natural blood flow, the oxygen supply, although great, cannot be increased to satisfy the work demands of the muscle. Moreover, the bending of the knees interferes with the circulation to the legs, making oxygen transport to the muscles quite difficult. Muscle twitchings also use much oxygen, adding to the oxygen debt.

EFFECTS ON THE HEART AND BLOOD VESSELS

AUSCULTATION

The auscultation of the heart revealed a rapid heart rate but no evidence of any murmurs, gallops, or other rhythm abnormalities, except that extrasystoles (missed beats) were heard on occasion. In some thin individuals, the heart was literally thumping against the chest wall.

BLOOD PRESSURE

When an individual's blood pressure is reported, two values are given, one high and one low. the high one is the systolic pressure, or the pressure in the arteries during contraction of the heart, and the low one is the diastolic pressure, or resting blood pressure in the arteries. A diastolic pressure above 90 and a systolic pressure above 140 is considered to be hypertension. The blood pressure increased during suspensions in all individuals tested, but the maximal response was variable from person to person and appeared related to the level of physical conditioning. For example, in one individual, the blood pressure rose from a resting pressure of 130/76 to 250/92 after five minutes, then dropped to 200/90, where it remained for up to fifteen minutes. Another individual had a resting blood pressure of 140/84 that rose to 168/92 after seven and a half minutes and remained at that pressure during the entire experiment. It is of significance that the diastolic pressure was above 90 in all of the individuals. The continued rapid heart rate is easily explained by this increased diastolic blood pressure, because when this pressure is increased in the heart, it becomes less responsive to the impulses that stimulate the vagus nerve, which decreases the heart rate. The blood pressure increases because of the increased output of the heart reflected by the increase in heart rate.

ELECTROCARDIOGRAPHIC MONITORING

The EKGs revealed marked muscular tremors due to the muscle twitching, but there was no evidence of any major abnormality indicative of lack of oxygen to the heart or rhythm abnormalities, except for an occasional bout of sinus tachycardia (rapid heart beat) in some individuals.

CARDIAC OUTPUT

The pulse rate increased progressively in all of the volunteers, but the degree of increase was variable. In most individuals, as in the blood pressure response, the degree of rise was dependent on the physical conditioning of the volunteers. In the instances where an individual was poorly conditioned, the pulse rate went up as high as 175 in the first two minutes. This was also influenced by the psychological state of the individual, with excitement causing release of adrenalin, according to the "fight or flight" reaction, as explained in the chapter on the sweating of blood. In these individuals, fear of the procedure caused a marked increase in pulse rate, but in subsequent hangings, the increase was significantly less because of their conditioning. The increased heart rate during the suspension procedure, therefore, is due to the release of adrenalin from the stress and the effects of muscle contractions and twitchings caused by carbon dioxide release, the increase in temperature, and the presence of diaphragmatic breathing, which in the early stages is somewhat insufficient but becomes very efficient with time.

BLOOD CHEMISTRIES

Blood samples were drawn before, during, and after hanging for the determination of lactic acid (explained previously), glutamic oxaloacetic transaminase (SGOT), glutamic pyruvic transaminase (SGPT), lactic dehydrogenase (LDH), creatinine phosphokinase

(CPK), isoenzymes of CPK and LDH. There was a two and a half times increase in the SGOT, a five times increase in the CPK from skeletal muscle, a slight increase in LDH, and no increase in the SGPT at twelve minutes, thirty-five seconds. This increase is a reflection of the marked skeletal muscle activity caused by the muscle contractions and twitchings and is not an indication of cardiac muscle damage because the heart isoenzymes of CPK showed no rise. The arterial blood cases were in the normal range.

RESULTS OF EXPERIMENTS

1. The angle of the arms with the upright varies between individuals with a wide range from sixty to seventy degrees.
2. At no time did the wrists change their angle when the volunteers were requested to push themselves up; instead the area naturally flexed at the elbows.
3. There was no visual evidence of breathing difficulties throughout the suspension.
4. Subjectively, every volunteer affirmed that they had absolutely no trouble breathing either during inspiration or expiration, in itself disproving the asphyxiation hypothesis.
5. A common complaint was a feeling of chest rigidity and leg cramps between ten and twenty minutes into suspension. When this occurred they were allowed to straighten their legs.
6. The oxygen content of the blood either increased or remained constant. Both visual observations and Douglas bag studies determined this to be the result of hyperventilation with abdominal breathing beginning after four minutes at a rate about four to five times normal.
7. Marked sweating occurred at about six minutes in most volunteers.
8. The heart rate increased up to 170 but there were no arrhythmias. There were occasional rapid rates as high as 175 but this went down after the volunteer got over the initial fright. The blood pressure increased to varying degrees in everyone depending on their state of conditioning. The electrocardiogram only showed muscle tremors and no cardiac abnormalities.
9. The backs of the volunteers never touched the cross except in the shoulder region where it was slight. Pain in the shoulders

caused many of them to arch their bodies back so that the top of the head touched the *stipes* thereby relieving some of the pain (Figure 9-4). None of the volunteers attempted to push up to facilitate breathing as suggested by Tribbe (1983) except when requested to do so.

CONCLUSION

The results of these studies overwhelmingly disprove the asphyxiation theory.

10

Miscellaneous

THE THIRST

"**A**fter this Jesus, knowing that all was now finished, said (to fulfill the Scriptures) 'I thirst.' A bowlful of vinegar stood there; so they put a sponge full of vinegar on hyssop and held it to his mouth. When Jesus had received the vinegar, he said, 'It is finished,' and he bowed his head and gave up his spirit" (John 19:28–30).

The desire for water to satisfy thirst is so basic to one's sense of survival that individuals have reacted both inappropriately and violently to such a degree that all sense of rationality ceases and survival becomes the all-encompassing mental focus.

The tortures associated with thirst are clearly envisioned in the article by LeBec (*Catholic Medical Guardian,* October 1925), who quoted an Arab scribe, el Sujuti, who in 1247 described a young Turk who was crucified in Damascus: "His worst agony was thirst. An eyewitness told me that he looked constantly from side to side imploring someone to give him a little water." McGee, an American geologist, who extensively studied the effects of thirst on individuals suffering from extremes of water deprivation in desert areas, distinguished five stages through which one passes on the way to death (as quoted by Dr. R. Whittaker in a paper read in 1935 before the St. Lukes Guild in London):

> In the first stage, there is a dryness of the mouth and throat accompanied by a craving for liquid. This is the common experience of normal thirst, and the condition may be alleviated, as ordinary practice shows, by a

102

moderate quantity of water or by exciting a flow of saliva in some way. In the second stage, the saliva and the mucous in the mouth and throat becomes sticky and scanty. There is a feeling of dry deadness of the mucous membranes. The in-breathed air feels hot and the tongue clings to the teeth and to the roof of the mouth. A lump seems to rise in the throat and starts endless swallowing motions in an attempt to dislodge it. Water and wetness are then exalted as the end of all excellence. Even in this stage, the distress can be alleviated by repeatedly sipping a few drops of water at a time.

We need not dwell on the last three stages described by McGee in which "the eyelids stiffen over the eyeballs set in a sightless stare, the tongue tip hardens to a dull weight, and the wretched victim has illusions of limpid pools and sparkling streams."

When Jesus said, "I thirst," there is no question that this was a gross underestimation. He had been deprived of liquid from the time of his last meal, which was the Last Supper the day before. Subsequently, he suffered the severe sweating of blood and water in the Garden of Gethsemane, the sweating and pleural effusion (fluid around the lungs) from the brutal scourging, the sweating from the pains of the crowning of thorns, carrying the cross, stripping his garments, and hanging on the cross. The pulmonary edema (fluid in the lung), pulmonary effusion, and edema of the extremities from hanging on the cross would certainly induce an agonizing thirst.

BLOOD AND WATER

"But one of the soldiers pierced his side with a spear and at once there came out blood and water" (John 19:34).

This phenomenon of blood and water has long been the subject of controversy, and many theories have been postulated in an attempt to explain it. To understand the various hypotheses and the validity of each, it behooves the reader to become familiar with the anatomy of the area to understand the mechanisms by which the body may form fluids around the lungs and chest.

The pericardium is a flask-shaped sac made up of a thin but very strong fibrous membrane that contains the heart and the roots of the great blood vessels, including the aorta (largest artery of the body, which conveys blood from the heart to all parts of the person), the vena cavae (which carries the blood back to the heart from the body), and the pulmonary artery and vein (which transports blood to and from the lungs). The pericardial sac is firmly anchored in the chest cavity with the neck of this sac closed around the great vessels located on the top of the heart. The base is strongly attached to the central part of the diaphragm (the thin, dome-shaped muscle that separates the chest cavity from the abdominal cavity), the sides of the sac are attached to each pleura (the membranes surrounding each lung), and the front of the sac is attached to the chest wall.

The heart, within the pericardial sac, extends over to the left side of the chest as is indicated in Figure 10-1. Note that the right atrium, which is the right upper chamber of the heart (labeled R. ATR.), extends about one inch to the right of the sternum (breastplate), while the left ventricle and right ventricle (the left lower chambers of the heart labeled LV and RV, as well as the left atrium or left upper chamber of the heart labeled L. ATR.) extend predominantly to the left side of the breastplate. If fluid accumulates in the pericardial sac, it is called *pericardial effusion,* a clear watery fluid, and if the blood accumulates in the pericardial sac, it is called *hemopericardium* and is usually due to a rupture of the heart muscle or of the root of the aorta. In a normal individual, the heart is relatively mobile within the sac, but in various pathological states, this mobility may be seriously compromised.

Each lung is also surrounded by a membranous sac called the pleura. The potential space between the pleura and the lung is called the *pleural space.* If fluid accumulates in this space from an injury (trauma) to the chest wall and lungs or from heart failure or other causes, it is called *pleural effusion* and consists of a clear, sometimes yellow-tinged, watery fluid. If blood accumulates in this space from an injury, it is called a *hemothorax.*

Now that we have a basic idea of the anatomy of this area and information regarding fluid or blood in the pericardial and pleural cavities, let us investigate and analyze the various hypotheses that have been put forth in an attempt to arrive at the most acceptable one.

In general, the water is either based on pleural or pericardial effusion from the scourging and/or from congestive heart failure caused by the position on the cross, from the separation of blood in the pleural or pericardial bottom layer, or from a bloody fluid in the pleural space caused by the scourging and/or heart failure that has separated out into an upper clear and bottom bloody layer.

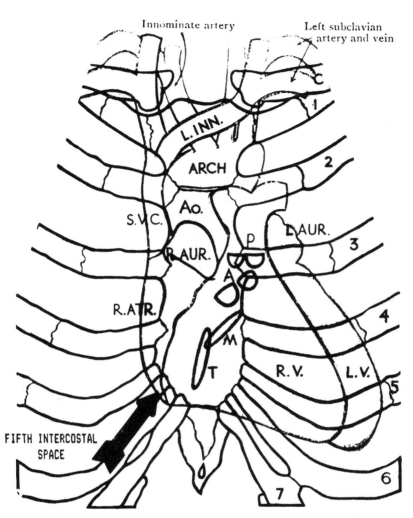

Innominate artery

Left subclavian
artery and vein

1 to 7. Ribs and costal cartilages.
  A. Aortic orifice.
 Ao. Ascending aorta.
  C. Clavicle.
L.V. Left ventricle.

M. Mitral orifice.
P. Pulmonary orifice.
R.V. Right ventricle.
S.V.C. Superior vena cava.
T. Tricuspid orifice.

<u>Figure 10-1</u>

Diagram of chest region.
This shows the relation of the heart and great vessels to the chest wall and ribs. The arrow (inserted by author) designates the proposed site where the spear entered the chest cavity.
(Courtesy of Oxford University Press, Oxford, England, from Cunningham's Manual of Practical Anatomy, vol. 2, figure 40.)

The presence of blood is explained by hemopericardium from a ruptured heart or ruptured aorta, hemoperitoneum from laceration of an abdominal artery, or separation of a bloody pleural effusion into an upper clear and lower bloody fluid from the scourging.

The hypotheses in general are divided into two major categories (see Table 10-1). Category 1 assumes that Christ was alive at the time that the spear pierced his side, and category 2 assumes that he was already dead.

There is no doubt that Jesus was dead at the time of the spear thrust because the scriptural account is clear on this point. St. John states, "So the soldiers came and broke the legs of the first and of the others who had been crucified with Him, but when they came to Jesus and saw that He was already dead, they did not break His legs, but one of the soldiers pierced His side with a spear and at once there came out blood and water" (John 19:32–34). All of the hypotheses supposing that Jesus was alive at the time of the spear thrust appeared to be based on the supposition that blood does not flow from a dead body. This is unfortunately false because blood does flow from a dead individual, particularly if death occurs violently. Certain chemical factors in the blood, responsible for clotting, do not appear to be particularly active in some persons, and a chemical substance, thrombolysins, which has the ability to dissolve clots, appears to be present in large amounts in such individuals. It has been my experience that blood remains unclotted in most individuals brought to autopsy within eight hours after death even in most cases due to natural causes. There appears to be some type of interference with blood clotting after death in these individuals. In victims of homicide, such as stabbings and gunshot wounds, as well as automobile accident victims, there is an oozing from the wounds during transport and other movements of the body.

The two theories based on the supposition that Christ suffered a rupture of the heart (Theories 1–5, Table 10-1) are both based on the supposition that Jesus died of a ruptured heart (cardiac tamponade).

Theory 7 (Table 10-1) also proposes a ruptured aorta, but with separation of the blood in the pericardial sac into an upper clear serum layer and a lower bloody layer, which is also not acceptable for two reasons. In all of the cases of cardiac tamponade that I have autopsied, on no occasion was a clear separation manifested. Second, the spear thrust would cause immediate mixing of the small volume of clear fluid, particularly if no clotting had occurred. Moreover, if clotting did occur, then there would be no blood for active flow, and only a light blood-tinged serum would extrude.

The thesis that the spear pierced the pericardial sac containing pericardial effusion as a result of the scourging (Theory 8, Table 10-1), proposed by Barbet, Judica-Cordiglia, and others, is also unacceptable. Even posttraumatic (injury) effusion, which measures twenty-five to fifty cubic centimeters, is too small in volume and would be immediately mixed with the blood from the right atrium of the heart as a consequence of the piercing action of the spear. I attempted to remove blood from the right atrium with a long needle for our routine toxicological analysis through the unopened pericardial sac in several cases of traumatic pericarditis with pleural effusion and noted that the fluid became bloody in a matter of seconds after removing the needle. There is no way that a clear fluid would flow from the pericardium to the chest wall through the "tunnel," as indicated by Barbet, without being admixed with blood.

The theory proposed by Primose, regarding abnormal effusion (fluid in the abdominal cavity) and piercing of the small vessels in the cavity, is also unacceptable (Theory 9, Table 10-1) because if a small vessel was pierced by the spear, it would almost immediately be admixed with the abdominal effusion fluid by the action of pulling out the spear, affording a pink fluid that certainly could not be interpreted as blood and water. It is also of interest that this hypothesis would be completely contrary to the evidence of the wound on the right side of the Turin Shroud (see Chapter 12).

The only two acceptable hypotheses are the last two listed (Theories 10 and 11, Table 10-1). Theory 10, which has been proposed by Savio, indicates that hemorrhagic effusion resulting from the brutal scourging settled into an upper clear layer and bottom bloody layer. When the spear pierced the chest wall, the blood extruded first, followed by the watery fluid. This theory appears possible, has probable merit, and must be considered as a possibility. The difficulty I have with this theory derives from the strong possibility that the fluid should be totally mixed when the spear pierces the cavity and is removed due to a mixing of both layers.

The last theory (Theory 11) indicates that the spear pierced the right atrium of the heart, hence the blood. The "water" resulted from the pleural effusion from the brutal scourging and was contributed to by congestive heart failure from the position on the cross. The sudden thrust of the spear with a quick, jerking motion to pull it out would certainly bring blood out first on the spear and would be followed immediately by the pleural effusion from the pleural cavity. I submit that the only blood flow after death in-cluded a small amount of a watery discharge containing blood that extruded from the lance wound. It is also important to realize that for a significant period of time prior to death, there would be very little blood flow from the wounds because the shock state would have caused marked hypotension. The amount of watery effusate and blood per se from the lance would have been small because the introduction of the spear would have immediately caused collapse of the lung due to the increased atmospheric pressure. Conse-quently, the fluid level would have dropped immediately because the lung volume after collapse is drastically decreased. The only watery fluid and blood flowing out of the wound would be due to the initial penetration by the lance (immediately prior to collapse) and small amount of blood from the right atrium of the heart contained on the spear tip by a quick, jerking motion after the sudden thrust. Many individuals have suggested that the intercostal spaces (spaces between ribs) are too small for a spear to enter far enough to penetrate the heart and that the heart, being relatively mobile, would slip aside. This is certainly not true because the rib spaces are variable from individual to individual and may be anywhere from one-half inch to a full inch wide. This provides adequate space for the Roman spear (the pilus), which has a small blade. Moreover, the thrust of the spear, even in individuals with small intercostal spaces, will easily pass through. I have seen numerous stab wounds of the heart made at various angles that would not compare with the force that could have been exerted with a Roman spear.

The ribs would readily spread apart from such force and momentum. Surgical operations on the chest cavity use an instru-ment called a rib spreader that easily spreads the space between ribs quite widely after an intercostal incision is made. The second objection, that the heart, being mobile, would push aside, making puncture difficult, is completely inconsistent with many cases of stabbing that I have investigated. The use of a spear would make puncture even more probable because of the longer handle and greater force.

TABLE 10-1
PROPOSED HYPOTHESES

I *Jesus Was Alive at Time of Spear Thrust*

THEORY 1
  (a) side pierced by spear
  (b) spear struck an artery of the chest wall (blood)
  (c) pleural effusion (fluid in chest cavity) due to scourging and/or congestive failure (water)

THEORY 2
  (a) heart pierced by spear (blood)
  (b) pleural effusion due to scourging and/or congestive failure (water)

THEORY 3
  (a) pericardial sac contained pericardial effusion due to scourging and/or congestive failure pierced by spear (water)

II *Jesus Was Dead at Time of Spear Thrust*

THEORY 4
  (a) pericardial sac pierced by spear contained blood (hemopericardium) under pressure from ruptured heart (blood)
  (b) pleural effusion due to scourging and/or congestive failure (water)

THEORY 5
  (a) pericardial sac pierced by spear contained blood from ruptured heart under pressure where blood had separated out into an upper clear serum layer (water) and bottom bloody layer (blood)

THEORY 6
  (a) pericardial sac pierced by spear contained blood under pressure from ruptured aorta (blood)
  (b) pleural effusion due to scourging and/or congestive failure (water)

THEORY 7
  (a) pericardial sac pierced by spear contained blood from ruptured aorta under pressure where blood had separated out into an upper clear serum layer (water) and bottom bloody layer (blood)

THEORY 8
  (a) pericardial sac contained an effusion from the scourging and/or congestive failure (water) and right atrium of heart (blood), both pierced by spear

THEORY 9
  (a) abdominal cavity on the left contained accumulation of fluid from scourging (water) and small blood vessel in cavity (blood), both pierced by spear

THEORY 10
> (a) side of chest pierced by spear contained hemorrhagic pleural effusion from scourging where blood had separated out into an upper clear serum layer (water) and bottom bloody layer (blood)

THEORY 11
> (a) right atrium of heart pierced by spear (blood) and pleural effusion from scourging and/or congestive failure (water)

REMOVING THE VICTIM FROM THE CROSS

The mechanism of removal was most logically the reverse of raising. The nails through the feet would be removed first. If the nail protruded through the back of the cross, it could be easily removed with a slight tap on the point end because it is wedge-shaped; otherwise, it would have to be gouged or chiseled out. The nail found through the heels of the crucified man in the Giv'at ha Mivtar excavation was bent at the point and still had a piece of the wood of the cross attached, confirming a chiseling or gouging technique of removal.

There are two possibilities for removing the hands. The *patibulum* could be lifted off by two individuals while one or two individuals grasped the victim around the waist. He would then be carried down the step device and the nails removed as indicated above. The second possibility, which appears very practical, requires that a rope be placed around the trunk, crossed at the back of the body (remember that during suspension the back is away from the upright), thrown over the crosspiece, and held taut by one or two men while the nails were removed as indicated above for the feet.

DID JESUS DIE OF A RUPTURED HEART OR HEART ATTACK?

There has been a recent interest in the hypothesis that attributes the death of Jesus to a rupture of his heart. This theory was alluded to by St. Bridgit, a mystic and the patron saint of Sweden, who revealed it after a vision of the crucifixion at an early age during the beginning of the fourteenth century. But it was not until 1874 that an Edinburgh physician named William Stroud first advanced the ruptured heart theory in his *Treatise on the Physical*

Cause of the Death of Christ, where he postulated that after the heart ruptured, the blood flowed into the sac surrounding the heart, called the pericardium, where the blood separated out into serum (water) and blood clot after death. In 1935, Dr. Ryland Whittaker, a Jesuit priest and physician, wrote in support of Stroud's theory because he was of the opinion that it was the only theory that could explain how the blood and water extruded from Christ's side. The most recent hypothesis of a ruptured heart was presented at the 1978 Second International Congress of the Shroud in Science in Turin, Italy, by Professor Ugo Wedessow, from the University of Milan in Italy, who postulated that Christ could very well have had a myocardial infarction several hours before he died, aggravated by the tortures he underwent. Before attempting to refute this hypothesis, it is necessary to understand the mechanism of spontaneous rupture of the heart.

The heart muscle receives its oxygen and nutrients through two blood vessels that encircle the heart like a crown, hence the term left and right coronary arteries. If one of these arteries becomes blocked or critically obstructed so that oxygen and nutrient-bearing blood cannot get through, areas of the heart beyond the blockage or occlusion will die and a heart attack will ensue. The area of heart muscle (myocardium) that dies is called an infarction, thus, a myocardial infarction is the synonym for a heart attack (Figure 10-2). The cause of blockage in a heart attack is almost always a condition called atherosclerosis, a type of arteriosclerosis (hardening of the arteries). This is a disease process in which a fatty substance is deposited on the arterial wall, thereby progressively narrowing the passage. Another way that myocardial infarction with subsequent rupture of the heart might occur is following severe injury (trauma) to the chest. During the week or so following a heart attack, after blockage or following injury to the myocardium, a process of softening occurs, making the heart muscle in the area of infarction particularly prone to rupture, and blood would flow under pressure into the sac surrounding the heart. This is referred to as cardiac tamponade. Rupture of the heart muscle occurs about seven days after a myocardial infarction, although there have been very rare instances of it occurring as early as one to two days after a massive infarction.

The theory of rupture of the heart as the cause of the death of Jesus would be untenable because of his age and the period of time in which death occurred. It would be extremely unlikely that Jesus

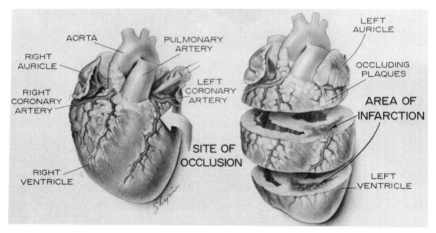

Figure 10-2
Diagram of the heart depicting a myocardial infarction (heart attack).
If one of the coronary arteries becomes obstructed, the heart muscle is deprived of
oxygen and nutrients and a myocardial infarction results.

suffered a heart attack because he was only thirty-three years of age,
and heart attacks were extremely rare in that region at the time of
Christ. When they did occur, it was in elderly individuals. Moreover, he would have had to have suffered the heart attack from one
to two days (which is extremely rare) to two weeks before his death.
Scriptures relate nothing regarding an illness prior to the sufferings
of Christ, and if Christ had a myocardial infarction in the Garden
of Gethsemane caused by the severe stress, we would have to
assume that he had severe occlusive disease of his coronary arteries
due to atherosclerosis, and, even then, the time following the
infarction would be insufficient for softening of the heart muscle to
occur. Even if the brutal scourging across the chest caused injury to
the heart severe enough to promote a heart attack by compromising
the circulation to the heart muscle, there would be insufficient
time for the heart muscle to attain the state that would cause it to
rupture. Therefore, the ruptured heart hypothesis should be dis-
carded and relegated to the archives of unfounded hypotheses
because it is totally unacceptable from a medical and scientific
point of view.

11

The Cause of Christ's Death

SHOCK—GENERAL CONSIDERATIONS

There is little doubt that *Jesus died as a consequence of shock.* To understand the mechanism of death in this manner, it is necessary to become familiar with the major types of shock.

Shock, by definition, is a condition where the blood flow to the tissues of the body is markedly reduced, causing a lack of oxygen and nutrients to them. Certain initiating factors cause a reduction of circulatory blood volume, which in turn causes a diminished venous return to the heart, which in turn decreases the output of blood by the heart, reducing blood flow to the tissues. The types of shock that we are concerned with include traumatic shock, hypovolemic shock, and cardiogenic shock.

Traumatic shock (injury shock) may be a consequence of physical injury to tissues even without a significant hemorrhage, where the presence of pain stimulates certain nervous mechanisms of the brain, resulting in a drop in blood pressure, ergo a reduction of blood flow to the tissues. The individual becomes ashen in color, lightheaded or dizzy, and breaks out in a sweat. It is common to find a person in shock following severe injuries even when there is no blood loss. It is the pain that induces the shock state, and an injection of an analgesic (painkiller), if given early, may dramatically prevent this state. I recall a case of an individual who was

113

trapped in a cave-in, requiring several hours to dig him out. He had excruciating pain and was becoming "shocky" when I arrived at the scene. I injected an analgesic and monitored his vital signs, such as blood pressure and pulse. All during the extrication procedure he remained out of shock.

Hypovolemic shock (low volume shock) is the type of shock where there is a marked fall in the blood volume due to hemorrhage or a loss of body water and electrolytes causing a drop in blood pressure, constriction (pinching off) of the peripheral (outside) blood vessels, and an increased heart rate in an attempt to compensate.

Cardiogenic shock (shock of the heart) occurs when there is a failure of the heart as a pump so that the output of blood by the heart is markedly reduced and blood backs up behind the heart so that there is an increase in venous pressure. This type of shock may occur following the two types of shock previously described, or as a complication of myocardial infarction (heart attack), certain rhythm disturbances of the heart, or congestive heart failure.

HOW DID SHOCK CAUSE THE DEATH OF JESUS?

In order to arrive at the most probable cause of death, it is essential to examine the sequence of all the events from Gethsemane through Calvary. The severe mental anguish exhibited in the Garden of Gethsemane would cause some loss in fluid volume from the circulation (hypovolemia) both from sweating and hematidrosis and would provoke marked weakness. The barbaric scourging that utilized a flagrum composed of leather tails containing metal weights or bone at the tip would cause penetration of the skin with trauma to the nerves, muscles, and skin, reducing the victim to an exhausted, wretched condition experiencing excruciating pain throughout his body, shivering, severe sweating, frequent displays of seizures, and a craving for water. The results would be a degree of traumatic (injury) shock and hypovolemia, the latter resulting from the sweating and the early stage of fluid around the lungs (pleural effusion) from the effects of the beating. Animal experimentation by Daniels and Cate showed that blows to the chest in animals resulted in rupture of the air spaces in the lung (alveoli) and spasm of the air tubes (bronchi). Moreover the term "traumatic wet lung" refers to the accumulation of blood, fluid, and mucus from severe trauma (injury) to the chest. The conclusion of traumatic shock from scourging was also made by both Tenney and Primrose. The irritation of the trigeminal and greater occipital nerves of the scalp by the cap of thorns from the Syrian Christ Thorn plant, *Zizziphus spina christ,* especially after he was struck several times with reeds, would cause lancinating pains, the worst type to which man is heir, across the scalp and face. These pains may have stopped intermittently only to begin again, more devastating each time he was struck with a scepter, or fell on his way to Calvary, and every time they pushed and shoved him. This would add to the state of traumatic shock induced by the scourging. The bumpy, uphill road to Golgotha in the hot sun, with the crosspiece on the shoulder for a time, with falling some of the time, and being struck other times also added to the hypovolemia and traumatic shock. Pleural effusion (water around the lungs) would gradually increase following the brutal scourging and begin to compromise breathing with shortness of breath. The consequences would be increasing hypovolemia. Concomitantly, the effects of scourging would now begin to manifest themselves with splinting of the chest wall (taking only shallow breaths to avoid movements of the ribs that cause severe pain each time the lungs are inflated) resulting in increasing hypovolemia. The large, square, iron nails driven through both hands into the cross would damage the sensory branches of the median nerve resulting in one of the most horrific pains ever experienced, known medically as *causalgia.* The nails through the feet would also elicit severe pain. Both of these would cause additional traumatic shock and hypovolemia. The hours on the cross, with pressure of the weight of the body on the nails present through the hands and feet would cause episodes of excruciating agony every time the *cruciarius* moved. These episodes and the unrelenting pains of the chest wall from the scourging would greatly worsen the state of traumatic shock, and the excessive sweating induced by the ongoing trauma and by the hot sun, would cause a greater degree of hypovolemic shock.

The pathophysiological events leading to death that occur as a result of these events are those of traumatic and hypovolemic shock. Shock, regardless of its cause is defined ". . . as a constellation of syndromes all characterized by low perfusion and circulatory insufficiency, leading to an imbalance between the metabolic needs of vital organs and the available blood flow"

(Robbins and Cotran, 1979, p. 183). It is "a state of inadequate perfusion of all cells and tissues, which at first leads to reversible hypoxic injury, but if sufficiently protracted or grave, to irreversible cell and organ injury and sometimes to the death of the patient" (Robbins, Cotran and Kumar, 1984, p. 112).

During crucifixion, there occurred certain attempts at compensation to the early phases of the shock by nerve and chemical influences to constrict blood vessels and increase heart rate, thereby causing an increase in blood pressure and output by the heart in an attempt to sustain adequate perfusion and oxygenation of vital organs. There were also compensatory mechanisms that caused the kidneys to conserve the plasma volume and promoted a shift of fluid from the capillaries into the main vessels. Immobilization of the body in the upright position caused hypostatic circulatory failure because the return circulation from the lower extremities through the veins was greatly dependent on gravity and the effects of muscular contraction after the blood was pumped by the heart to these areas. With this progressive development of spaces, because of the bending of the knees and transfixing of the hands and feet to the cross, the organs, such as the liver and kidney, became engorged with blood.

During the time of suspension there was a progressive loss of plasma to the pleural spaces and to the tissue spaces such as the ankles, pooling of blood to the lower parts of the body from the position on the cross, and continued sweating caused by the direct rays of the hot midday sun, the heat produced by the increased muscular activity, and the hypotensive (low blood pressure) responses of the body to pain. Because there was no attempt to replace the lost fluids or to stop the pain, the compensatory mechanisms reached their saturation point.

This presents a very complex array of initiating factors, compensatory reactions and several interrelationships much too complex to include here. In this regard the reader is referred to my article "Death by Crucifixion" published in the *Canadian Society of Forensic Sciences Journal*, 1983, for an in-depth discussion of the mechanisms of shock invoked during crucifixion, from initiation to death. In the interest of truth, I presented my research findings and conclusions, the asphyxiation theory, and the ruptured heart theory in a paper entitled, "Death by Crucifixion" before the Forensic Pathology Section at the 35th Annual Meeting of the American Academy of Forensic Sciences in Cincinnati, Ohio, on 19 February

1984, which is considered to be one of the most critical and prestigious forums in forensic pathology in the world.

The paper was well received and many pathologists indicated that they concurred with my conclusions. Not a single pathologist present challenged my findings or conclusions.

Writing in *Sindone,* Drs. Angelino and Abrate concluded that death in crucifixion is due to traumatic and hypovolemic shock, and Dr. William Edwards, from the Mayo Clinic, recently implicated hypovolemia as a cause of death in crucifixion, which he reported in the *Journal of the American Medical Association.* After reading my study, Dr. Alan Adler informed me that his findings of elevated biliary substances on the Shroud supported the conclusion that death was due to shock.

It is also of interest to note that Barbet included the opinion of the surgeon P. J. Smith, in Appendix II (page 175) of his book, *Doctor at Calvary.* Dr. Smith disagreed with Barbet about the cause of death. He states

> I am of the opinion that there is overwhelming evidence that Christ died from heart failure due to extreme shock caused by exhaustion, pain and loss of blood. Asphyxia, or respiratory failure as we prefer to call it, the author thinks was caused by the respiratory muscles becoming fixed in inspiration due to the falling forward of the trunk away from the vertical section of the cross and the consequent ability to expire and so empty the lungs of carbon dioxide. This theory is not supported by some of the evidence set out in the book.

THE CAUSE OF DEATH OF JESUS

The death certificate in this case, if signed today, would read somewhat as follows:

Cardiac and Respiratory Arrest Due to Hypovolemic and Traumatic Shock Due to Crucifixion

WHY DID JESUS DIE SO SOON?

"Joseph of Arimathea, a respected member of council, who was also himself looking for the Kingdom of God, took courage and went to Pilate and asked for the body of Jesus. And Pilate wondered if he were already dead and summoned the centurian, he asked him whether he was already dead. And when he learned from the centurion that he was dead, he granted the body of Jesus" (Mark 15:43–45).

Pilate seemed surprised that Jesus died so soon, and certainly this was based on his vast experience in the many crucifixions that he had ordered. The reason for the apparent rapid demise of Jesus derives primarily from the fact that, unknown to Pilate, Jesus was already in an exhausted state from his severe mental sufferings in the Garden of Gethsemane prior to the terrible scourging. The significance of mental suffering is not frequently realized unless one understands that it relentlessly saps the strength of an individual to a state of total exhaustion. Moreover, Pilate's intention during the scourging, as stated previously, was to reduce Jesus to a wretched state in order to avoid crucifixion because he merely wanted to appease the mob. Therefore, Jesus was severely flogged, greatly exceeding the number of lashes normally used as a prelude to crucifixion. Add this effect to the mental anguish, the scourging, and the crowning of thorns, to the effects of carrying the cross and the crucifixion process, and anyone with a medical background cringes and wonders conversely how he lasted as long as he did and certainly would not be in the least surprised that he was already dead.

12

A Medical Examiner Interprets the Turin Shroud

TURIN, ITALY—AUGUST 27–OCTOBER 8, 1978

When we arrived on Wednesday, October 4, Turin was bustling with crowds of pilgrims (Figures 12-1 and 12-2). Three million in all had visited this city during a six-week period from August 27 to October 8. They were here to see the Shroud, known as the Sindone of Turin, a relic extraordinaire, the cloth believed to have wrapped the body of Jesus after his removal from the cross, and bearing an image of the entire body front and back of Jesus the crucified (Figure 12-30). This was the first public exposition since 1933, the result of the diplomatic efforts of Father Peter Rinaldi, a Salesian priest, who has dedicated most of his life to the study of the Shroud. All day long, pilgrims stood in a line that appeared to be about one-half mile in length and about eight people in width (Figure 12-2), continuing at a relatively steady pace, and requiring from three to four hours to obtain a glimpse of the Holy Shroud in the Shroud Chapel of St. John the Baptist, known as the Duomo (Cathedral of San Giovanni Battista).

I saw the Shroud early Saturday morning, October 7, displayed high above the altar in a frame protected with bullet-proof glass because of previous attempts to destroy the relic (Figure 13-2). It was a mystifying experience to behold the image on the Shroud after so many years, twenty-five in all, of studying the photographs

119

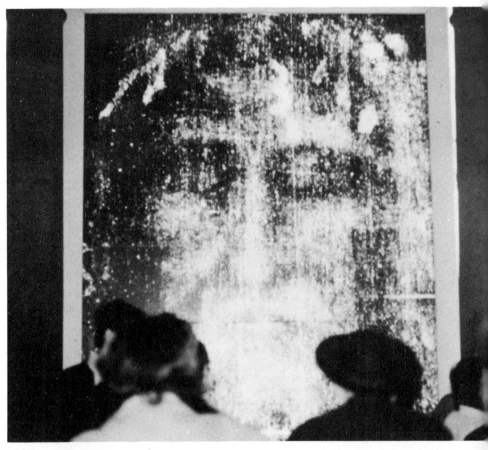

Figure 12-1
Giant posters of Shroud.
Turin, Italy, during Exposition of 1978.

taken by Enrie. Although I was only a few feet away from the Shroud, I used a pair of exquisite quality Zeiss 8 × 30 wide-angle binoculars to observe certain fine details of the wounds of the hands and the imprints of the feet.

The last two days of the exposition on October 7 and 8 were reserved for the Second International Scientific Conference of Sindonology to which I was extended the privilege of participating (Figure 12-1). It was held at the Instituto Bancario San Paolo on the Piazza Giorgio Cavallo, magnificent rector of the University of

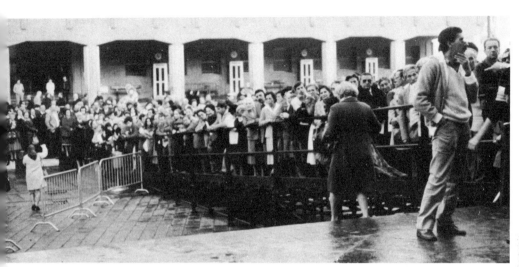

Figure 12-2
Pilgrims in line to see the Shroud.
Italy, during Exposition of 1978. The lines were about eight persons wide and about a mile long, from early morning to late evening.

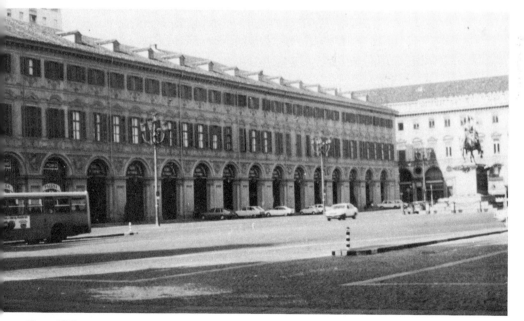

Figure 12-3
Instituto Bancario San Paola.
Piazza San Carlo in Turin. Site of Second International Conference of Sindonology, 1978.

Turin. Scientists interested in this subject came from throughout the world and represented the fields of pathology, biology, electronics, thermonuclear physics, palinology, criminalistics, anatomy, surgery, computer studies, textile archaeology, art history, radiology, chemistry, and nuclear physics. They were here to present their findings, exchange new ideas, and discuss recent developments.

The week following this conference had been cleared for one hundred and twenty hours of scientific studies of the Shroud. Activities included visible, ultraviolet and infrared spectroscopy, light, ultraviolet and phase microscopy, infrared thermography, x-radiographic imaging, electron microscopy, computer analysis, photographic imaging with special films, microchemical analysis, etc.

THE SHROUD—GENERAL CONSIDERATIONS

The Turin Shroud or sindone is a long, winding linen sheet that measures 14'3" (4.3 meters) in length and is 3'7" (1.1 meters) in width. The linen is irregularly woven in a herringbone pattern and appears worn in places. A mystifying image, front and back, of a crucified individual, believed to be that of Jesus Christ, is portrayed in variable, diffuse tones of a pale, brownish-yellow color that appears more distinct at a distance and fades out when viewed at different angles, particularly as one comes closer to the Shroud. Areas representing blood from various wounds made by nails, scourging, the crown of thorns, and the spear were more vividly seen in a deeper color resembling puce (Figure 10-1).

In 1898, a lawyer, Secondo Pia, who was also an amateur photographer, was afforded the honor of photographing the Turin Shroud during an exposition to honor the marriage of the future king, Victor Emmanuel III. He had only two tries to accomplish this feat in between the various visits by the pilgrims. The first attempt on May 25 met with failure because he broke his emery filters and the illumination proved unsatisfactory. But the second attempt on May 28 was victorious, in spite of the crystal glass that now had been ordered by Princess Clothilde and placed around the Shroud to prevent damage by candle smoke and incense. Pia took two exposures on fifty by sixty centimeter orthochromatic plates of fourteen minutes and twenty minutes, respectively, because of the slow film speed at that time. While developing the negative late at night, Pia noted that the negative afforded an astounding photograph of the image in unbelievable negative quality with a complete inversion of light values, giving the Shroud the characteristics of a true negative, and the actual negative the characteristics of a positive print (Figures 12-4 and 12-5). Pia was deeply moved and indicated that he experienced such an emotional impact when he first viewed the face that he remained almost frozen (Figure 3-4).

Giuseppe Enrie, editor of *Vita Photographica Italiana,* on May 3, 14, and 15, 1931, was enlisted to take the official photographs of the Shroud during the exposition in honor of the wedding of King Umberto II. He made a series of excellent photographs using the latest equipment and best photographic knowledge of the time. No retouching was done. In fact, several photographers brought in to examine the plates attested to the fact that they were not retouched, and an affidavit was filed before Turin notary Guilo Turbilo on May 28, 1931.

A front and back image occurs because the crucified individual was laid out on one end of the long, winding linen sheet that had been placed on the ground. The opposite end of the Shroud was then brought up over the top of his head over the face and down to the front of the body, as shown by the painting of G. Clovio, which has been reproduced by G. B. della Rovere and now hangs in the Galleria Sabauda Torino (Figure 12-6). The figure on the cloth has been estimated to be from 5'10½" to 6'2" tall. The body is naked, bearded, long-haired, with an image in the back extending to the shoulder blades resembling a pigtail. The right shoulder is lower than the left, and one foot appears turned in toward the other. There is no discernible neck space, and the hands are crossed just below the umbilicus at the hip level, with the left over the right (because the Shroud is in actuality a negative image, the left side of the body would be the right and vice versa). This crossing of the hands and position of the feet suggests that they were bound. A bifurcated, puce-colored image is present on the left hand between the wrist and the hand *per se* representing the nail wound. The face has a masklike appearance with the eyes presenting an owl-eyed look. In the frontal view, the forehead area shows a rivulet in the form of a backward figure 3 pattern in the center with other small streams on the left and right of the forehead and in the hair, all representing bleeding from the crown of thorns. The back of the head likewise shows an aggregation of similar dark red stains, also indicative of the results of the sharp thorns.

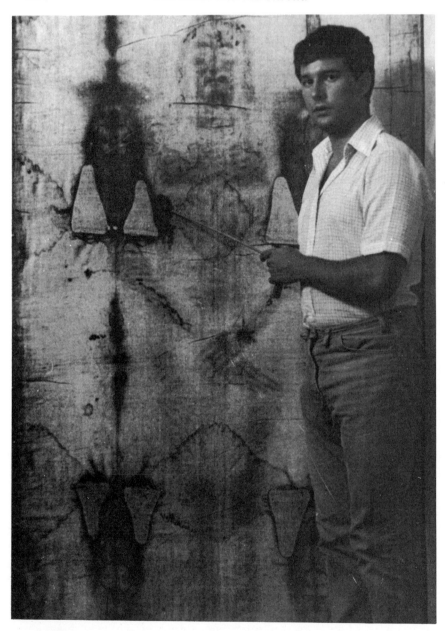

Figure 12-4

Shroud of Turin, full size frontal view as it appears to the viewer.
A print from the negative shown in Figure 12-5.
(Courtesy of Gene Hoyas).

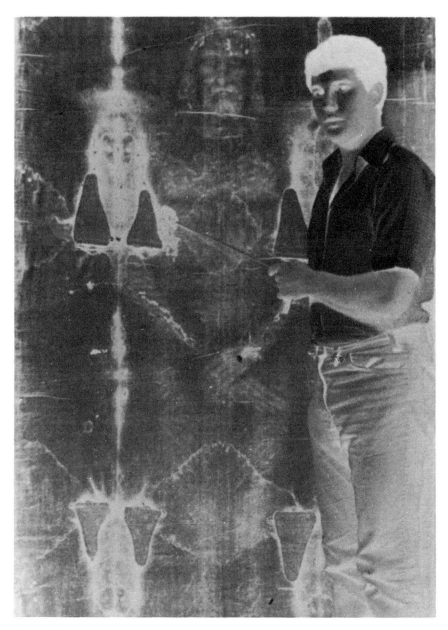

Figure 12-5
Shroud of Turin, full size frontal view as it appears on the negative film when photographed.
The Shroud shown in Figure 12-4 possesses all of the characteristics of a true photographic negative.
(Courtesy of Gene Hoyas.)

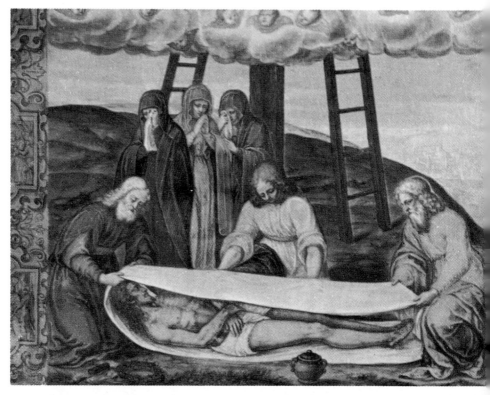

Figure 12-6
How the Shroud was wrapped.
Painting by Giovanni Battista della Rovere, a sixteenth-century artist, at the Galleria Sabauda.

The back, buttocks, legs, chest, and abdomen show evidence of a brutal scourging depicted as dumbbell-like images. Two images, in the region of the left shoulder blade and right back, suggest bruises that some individuals have related to carrying of the cross. The feet area reveals the right sole and heel and the left heel only and contains several images corresponding to the nailing of the feet. The right side of the body contains a large puce-colored image in the region corresponding to the fifth or sixth intercostal space, representing the wound from the spear, and deep reddish streams assuming multidirectional flows are noted on the arms.

There are two dark linear impressions with breaks on both sides of the Shroud with four double pairs of white triangular areas representing the results of the fire that occurred at the Sainte Chapelle de Chambéry on December 3, 1532. The Shroud was folded in a silver casket at that time, and some of the silver melted onto the Shroud, making the four holes in the center of the cloth at the level of the top of the head. The dark triangular areas, which are similar in color but darker than the images, represent the burns, the white triangular pairs are the patches sewn by the Poor Clares, and the dark lines are the burned areas of the folds. Large stains from the water used to put out the fire are vividly displayed.

BRIEF HISTORY OF THE SHROUD

A brief review of the history of the Turin Shroud is herein presented to give the reader a thumbnail sketch; a full historic account would be superfluous in view of the numerous excellent accounts now available (refer to list of references at the end of this book).

Historic documentation is firm as far back as 1349, when the Shroud was in the possession of Geoffrey de Charny, Lord of Lirey, but its history prior to this time has been the seat of much controversy. References to a Shroud or image are as follows: in the first two centuries, by the apocryphal gospels; in the fourth century by Arculfo, bishop of France; in the twelfth century by Louis VII and Emmanuel the first Comneno; and in the thirteenth century by Robert of Clary. The studies of the late Paul Vignon, professor of biology at the Institut Catholique in Paris, at the beginning of this century, gave great impetus to filling the gaps in chronology. He found that icons and other early paintings of the head of Jesus contained striking similarities to the image on the Turin Shroud, such as forked beard, absence of a neck, straight nose, one raised eyebrow, a divided mustache, staring eyes, wide nostrils, and peculiar markings consisting of a square, boxlike figure with the upper side missing and with or without a "V" below the box in the area between the eyes. The icons contained some or all of the above characteristics, the earliest of which dated back to about the sixth century (see Figure 12-7).

The recent scholarly studies by Ian Wilson, although quite circumstantial and speculative, indicate that the Shroud of Turin and the Image of Edessa, later referred to as the Mandylion, were one and the same. The legend of the Edessa image relates that King Abgar V of Edessa (now Turkey) was ill with leprosy and sent for

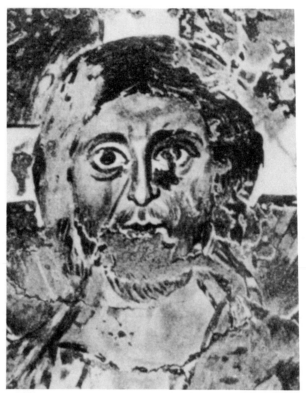

Figure 12-7
Icon of St. Pontianus.
Catacombs in Rome, sixth or seventh century.

Jesus to heal him. Instead, Jesus sent him a cloth containing a miraculous image of his face, which immediately cured him. The image was referred to as *archeiropoitos*, which in Greek is translated "not made with hands." Wilson developed the concept that the Edessa image was folded in fours with a backing and kept in a casket until the thirteenth century, when it appeared in Constantinople. In support of this, he demonstrated that if a full-length photograph of the Turin Shroud is folded in fours, it will show only the face. This implies that the Mandylion, or the Image of Edessa, was in reality the Shroud of Turin and allegedly was taken to France in the thirteenth century from Constantinople by a Knight Templar of the Charny family. The Knight Templars were a secret, religious order consisting of former crusaders who worshiped a mysterious image and who fought to protect the needy.

Geoffrey de Charny built the Lirey Church in the early 1350s at which time he installed the Shroud. It remained in the Chapel of Lirey until 1452 when Margaret de Charny, granddaughter of Geoffrey de Charny, traded the Shroud to Anna de Lusignano, wife of Ludovigo, duke of Savoy, for two castles. It was kept in Chambéry in a silver casket. In 1532, a fire broke out and melted part of the silver casket, causing the molten silver to burn the edges of the Shroud. This was repaired with patches by the Poor Clares. The Shroud traveled to Turin, Vercelli, Nice, and Chambéry during the French-English wars. In 1578, the Shroud was brought to Turin by Emmanuel Filbert to spare archbishop of Milan St. Charles Borromeo, the rigorous trip over the Alps. St. Charles made a pilgrimage on October 6, 1578, in fulfillment of a vow made during the ravages of the plague in Milan that he would venerate the Turin Shroud. The Shroud was placed in the Chapel of Guarini in 1694. In 1918, during World War I, it was transferred to a place of safety and again during World War II, on September 25, 1939, when it was ordered hidden in the Benedictine Monastery of the Montevergine in Avelion, northeast of Naples. The Shroud remained in a fortresslike structure until October 28, 1946, when it was re-

Figure 12-8

Italy hides Shroud.
The Shroud was safely hidden in a monastery northeast of Naples during World War II (see text.)

ITALY HIDES SHROUD OF CHRIST IN SAFER, SECRET REPOSITORY

[By Wireless to the New York Times and The Chicago Tribune.]

BERNE, Switzerland, April 2.— The Giornale d'Italia reported today that as a result of aerial bombardments the shroud in which Christ was buried and which has been preserved in the chapel of the cathedral of Turin has been taken secretly to a safe repository.

Only the king of Italy, the crown prince, and the archbishop of Turin know the spot to which the pall has been removed. Transfer was confirmed in a notarial deposition.

The genuineness of the relic, which in the course of history has been several times contested was established scientifically only 12 years ago.

turned to Turin (see newspaper clipping, Figure 12-8). An exposition of the Shroud took place in 1931 in honor of Umberto II of Savoy, King of Italy and owner of the Shroud, and again in 1933 in honor of the 1900-year anniversary of Christ's death and resurrection. Since its purchase in 1452 and until the death of Umberto II on March 18, 1983, the Shroud has been under the ownership of the House of Savoy. King Umberto II willed the Shroud to Pope John Paul II (see newspaper clipping, Figure 12-9).

SCIENTIFIC CONCEPTS AND POSTMORTEM INTERPRETATIONS

To interpret the Shroud in a more meaningful manner, it is necessary that the reader become familiar with certain concepts in forensic pathology, including rigor mortis, cadaveric spasm, and

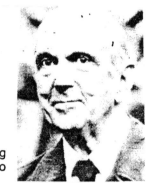

King
Umberto

Shroud of Turin Left to Pope

Italy's deposed **King Umberto**, who died March 18, left the Shroud of Turin, believed to be the burial cloth of Jesus Christ, to Pope John Paul II in his will, a spokesman for the family has confirmed.

The shroud, a 14-foot-long linen cloth, is on display to the public in the Turin cathedral, but has belonged to the royal house of Savoy since the Middle Ages. It bears marks many Catholics believe to be the imprint of the face of Christ.

Figure 12-9
Shroud of Turin left to Pope.
1983 newspaper clipping.

characteristics of postmortem blood. These concepts are very important because there is strong evidence that the "Man of the Shroud" was in the state of rigor mortis prior to being placed on the Shroud, and because the various imprints indicative of wounds and blood flow patterns require scientific interpretation.

RIGOR MORTIS

Rigor mortis is a stiffening and shortening of all of the muscles of the body after death caused by an irreversible chemical reaction. The jaws, neck, arms, legs, and trunk become almost rock hard and remain in the position the individual was in just prior to death. For example, if the individual died while one leg was propped in an elevated position or the arm was propped above his head, these limbs would remain that way after rigor mortis had set in. This fact has medico-legal significance to determine if a body had been moved after rigor mortis set in. For example, if a body was found lying flat with the legs suspended in the air, it would be immediately obvious that the body was moved from a position where the legs were resting on something. Rigor mortis usually begins in the jaw muscles about three hours after death and appears progressively in the muscles of the neck, chest, arms, and legs, becoming complete in about twelve to eighteen hours. The rigor state will usually remain for about twelve hours and gradually go away, leaving the body in the same sequence in twelve or more hours. Although rigor mortis is used in forensic pathology as a means of assessing the time of death, it is very variable, hence by no means reliable, and must be used with other criteria.

Rigor mortis is caused by a complex chemical reaction inherent to the muscle fibers. Each muscle is made up of microscopic myofibrils that are chemically made up of two types of protein filaments called actin and myosin filaments. During muscle contractions, these filaments interact with each other, causing a sliding of a rod of actin between rods of myosin, almost like the effect of a piston within a cylinder. A chemical of the body called adenosine triphosphate, known as ATP, which supplies energy to the muscle, becomes used up after death, and rigor mortis ensues.

This chemical reaction is modified by many factors. Production of heat, such as occurs with fever, warm weather, or increased muscular activity, stimulates the chemical reaction, causing more rapid rigor mortis, while cold retards it. I recall a case where an individual was shot after being chased down alleys and over fences for a long distance and developed almost immediate rigor mortis.

BREAKING THE RIGOR

If a person is in complete rigor mortis the only way to change the position of a limb at a joint is to *break the rigor*, a term referring to the forcible bending of a limb at any joint. For example, if an elbow is in rigor mortis and bent to an angle of forty-five degrees, straightening of the arm is possible by forcibly straightening it. The greater the muscular development, the greater the force required to break the rigor.

There is an indication that the man of the Shroud was in a state or rigor mortis when placed on the Shroud; the absence of a neck space in the front image and an elongated image on the back of the neck area is highly suggestive that the head was bent forward in rigor. The leg and foot images are also highly suspect of rigor mortis since the right calf shows a greater density than the left. And the left foot shows an imprint of only part of the heel suggesting either a very slight bend at the left knee with the foot flexed slightly forward or a turning inward of the left foot over the right (refer to Chapter 12, Feet). If rigor were not present there should be symmetrical images of the legs. Therefore, the man of the Shroud would have been fixed in an attitude of suspension. Moreover, when he was taken down from the cross, in addition to breaking the rigor at the knees, the rigor had to be broken at the shoulder joint and slightly at the elbows in order to assume the position present on the Shroud. Professor James Cameron, a well-known forensic pathologist at the London Hospital, also attributes the arm stiffness to rigor mortis and contends that those who took the body down from the cross had to forcibly break the rigor at the shoulders so the arms could be placed as they are shown on the Shroud.

DOES BLOOD FLOW AFTER DEATH?

The answer to the question of whether blood flows after death is of major importance in answering questions regarding the various blood patterns on the Shroud, as well as the explanation of the phenomenon of blood and water discussed previously. Blood after death may be in a clotted or unclotted state depending on the circumstances. In general, the works of Yudin (1937), in his review of five hundred cases, indicated that blood of individuals dying from severe diseases, such as cancer, tuberculosis, and sepsis, may be clotted and cannot be dissolved until putrefaction of the body occurs. In sudden or violent deaths, such as severe trauma, automobile accidents, electrocutions, concussions, and gunshot blasts, clotting initially may begin, but in a matter of fifteen minutes or one-half hour, the blood becomes fluid again. This is not a firm rule; we frequently see fluid blood in individuals with severe disease and coagulated blood in individuals following sudden or violent deaths, but only on rare occasions in the latter case. Studies by Mole (1948) revealed that the fluidity was related to the presence of fibrinolysins, which are chemicals formed in the body that dissolve blood clots. He found that their presence was associated with rapidity of death. Another factor of importance is that after postmortem blood flows from a wound, it rarely coagulates, but may dry. Any kind of moisture will reliquefy it.

In our daily experiences in the medical examiner's office, we commonly observe bleeding or oozing from lacerations, bullet wounds, stab wounds, traumatic injuries, and the like, even the next day when moving the body around in the autopsy room. In addition to the fluidity of the blood caused by the thrombolysins and altered clotting factors, there is an absence of the normal contractions of tiny blood vessels that play a prominent role in bleeding control in the living state.

The answer to the question whether blood might flow after death in the case of Jesus may now be answered in the affirmative because his death fulfills the criteria of a violent death that could lead to fluidity of the blood, and this coupled with an absence of contractions of the small blood vessels could easily account for many of the blood streams noted on the Shroud of Turin.

THE MAN OF THE SHROUD WAS WASHED AFTER DEATH

Imprints depicting the various wounds inflicted on the man of the Shroud include numerous dumbbell-shaped scourge marks over the trunk (Figures 2-3 and 12-14), an exact pattern of rivulets of blood on the left arm, a single tortuous flow of blood on the forehead, a precise bifurcation pattern on the back of the hand, and a small clump of blood on the heel. Ultraviolet light studies of these patterns are even more vivid in terms of preciseness; the scourge marks show well-defined borders, and fine scratchlike markings appear mingled in-between.

The controversy as to whether or not the man of the Shroud was washed prior to being placed on the burial cloth has far reaching significance in terms of authenticity of the Shroud of Turin. The concept that the crucified was not washed prior to being placed on the Shroud would not be readily acceptable by the forensic pathologist whose expertise includes studies of antemortem and postmortem blood flow patterns. Acceptance of the hypothesis that the crucified was not washed would therefore place the authenticity of the Turin Shroud in serious doubt.

THE SCOURGE WOUNDS

If the deceased individual had not been washed, these well-defined wound patterns depicted on the Shroud could not be present. First of all, most of the blood within the scourge wounds of the victim would have been clotted and the blood located both at the periphery and outside of the wounds would have dried long before the victim was placed on the cross. According to the experiments of Lavoie et al., a cloth would have to be placed on a moist clot no later than two and one half hours after bleeding stopped. In addition, these authors argue that moistened clots have to be transferred within an hour for a good mirror image transfer to take place. Forgetting all of the other wounds, no one would argue that the scourge wounds were made and clotting began several hours prior to death. Moreover, most forensic experts agree that the man of the Shroud shows evidence of rigor mortis as previously indicated in the section, Rigor Mortis, thus indicating that the crucified was dead for some time before being taken down from the cross. According to the studies of Lavoie's group, these *perfectly defined wounds* should not have transferred at all. Yet many of the scourge wounds on the Shroud of Turin are extremely distinct, corresponding to dumbbell-shaped wounds. Even if the clots from these wounds satisfied the time and moisture criteria postulated by Lavoie's group, the shape of the scourge wounds—including the bloody areas around the wounds—would be indistinct and extremely variable in size and shape depending on the depth and angle of the wound, the amount of blood flow, the flow pattern, and whether or not clothing adhered to the wounds. Moreover, even if the dripping sweat of the crucified softened some of the dried blood in areas just outside these wounds, only indistinct and variable-shaped impressions would result. However, if the body was washed, the dried blood around the wounds would be removed causing an oozing of bloody material within the wounds. This would result in the production of relatively good impressions of the wound. In order to test this hypothesis, at autopsy pieces of linen and paper towels were gently touched (not pressed) against wounds from accident victims who had lived for several hours following the accident. Relatively no impressions were made. This was repeated after the wounds were rinsed with water and allowed to soak on the wounds for several minutes. Only indistinct bloody impressions were made. The wounds were then washed and this procedure tried again. This resulted in reasonably good impressions of the wounds (Figure 12-10).

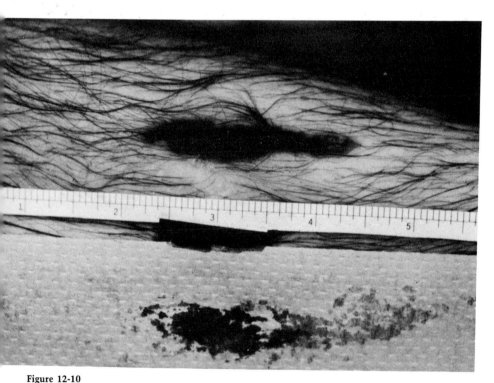

Figure 12-10
Impression of wound from auto accident.
At autopsy, several hours after accident. Top, wound prior to washing. Bottom, impression made after washing with water.

HAND WOUND

An excellent example of the lack of understanding regarding blood flow patterns derives from the so called double flow blood pattern presumed to represent two positions assumed by the crucified in order to breathe while on the cross, referred to as the asphyxiation or suffocation theory. After extensive experimentation, this theory was recently shown untenable. However, even if the asphyxiation hypothesis was found to be correct, logical reasoning from the forensic point of view precludes the acceptance of two distinctly defined flow patterns to signify the two presumed positions for breathing hypothesized by Barbet for the following reasons. First of all, the pattern is located on the *back* of the hand where it is compressed against the cross beam (*patibulum*) of the cross by nailing. Since the crucified's heart is beating, blood would constantly extrude from this area during every agonizing movement causing a large blood smudge around both the nail and the wound, all over the back of the hand, and probably down the arm. Moreover, even if the two well-defined blood flow patterns were located on the front of the wrist where smudging would not occur, they could not be attributed to the two alleged breathing positions because the blood flows would have run into each other causing a pooling of blood due to the various positions assumed by the crucified on the cross.

What then would account for the peculiar bifurcation pattern on the back of the hand? The most logical explanation for this pattern may be explained by the formation of rivulets of blood running to the two sides of the ulnar styloid protuberance (the bump on the back of the wrist on the little finger side) after removing the nail from the wrist, sometime after removal from the cross. A case in mind involved the homicidal shooting of a young man who received multiple gunshot wounds. During the autopsy, I noted the presence of two dried blood rivulets running from a gunshot wound located in the forearm just above the wrist to both sides of the ulnar styloid protuberance. I then realized that this gunshot wound was the one I had probed at the scene the evening before in an effort to determine the trajectory. This probing had disturbed the dried blood and the act of removal of the body by the morgue attendants from the scene to the medical examiner's office caused the blood to flow to this area. A similar mechanism would account for the bifurcation pattern of the hand wound on the

Shroud. In order to demonstrate flow patterns, wounds from accident victims who had lived for several hours following an accident were briefly washed at autopsy and observed for oozing of blood. Within a few minutes, a small rivulet of blood appeared (Figures 12-11 and 12-12).

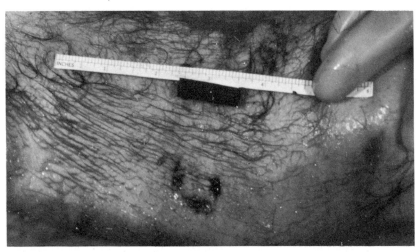

Figure 12-11
Wound from auto accident before washing.
At autopsy. Victim lived several hours after the accident.

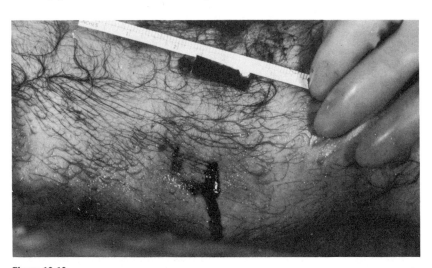

Figure 12-12
Wound from auto accident after washing.
Same wound as in Figure 12-11 after a gentle water wash. Note oozing with blood flow pattern after a few seconds.

There is another experiment supporting my contention that the bifurcation pattern of the hand wound could not be explained by a raising and dropping position of the crucified in order to breathe. Experiments using volunteers suspended on an accurate cross revealed a bending of the elbows with no change in the angle of the wrist when the volunteers attempted to raise their body. In the case of actual crucifixion, this would even be more striking since a square nail passing tightly through the tendinous areas between the bones of the wrist and then embedded into the *patibulum* would affix the hand and wrist solidly assuring no change in angle.

ROLE OF THE FORENSIC PATHOLOGIST

The expertise concerning blood flow patterns is in the area of forensic pathology. The forensic pathologist is frequently called in to court to provide expert testimony regarding blood flow patterns and wound characteristics and to render an opinion regarding the mechanism, manner, and cause of death concerning these circumstances. This applies to the man on the Shroud who was apparently scourged, crowned with thorns, nailed through the hands and feet with large square nails, and suspended by the hands for several hours. A forensic evaluation of the crucifixion reveals that every movement during the entire time the crucified was on the cross would have restarted bleeding in the hand and foot wounds. The body unquestionably would have been literally covered with blood because the heart pumps about 4,500 gallons of blood through the more than 60,000 miles of large and small blood vessels throughout the whole body each day. Instead of the very exact imprints of the wounds, the Shroud would bear large indistinct masses of blood over the entire image including the face, arms, hands, feet, and trunk. Studies by Adler showing the presence of blood only on the wound image areas, and not on the body-areas, only support this.

Every practicing forensic pathologist knows that even tiny wounds may bleed profusely during heart activity and observes the end results of bleeding from wounds of practically every type on a daily basis. It is also important to realize that for a significant period of time prior to death, there would be very little blood flow from the wounds because the shock state would have caused marked hypotension in the crucified individual. It is also of importance to note that scourge markings were made many hours prior to removal from the cross so that encrusted clots would have formed in the wounds therefore making it difficult to understand how the scourge marks could have left such precise imprints. Every forensic pathologist I have consulted agreed that the wounds would have caused a large amount of bleeding and that the body had to be washed to account for the preciseness of the wounds. And in the December 1980 issue of *Medical World News*, Dr. Michael Baden, a forensic pathologist and the former chief medical examiner of New York City, agreed that if the Shroud is genuine, the body must have been washed. He also added that if the body was washed there might be some oozing from the wounds.

An observation of major importance that supports the washing hypothesis was reported by Jumper et al. in *Archaeological Chemistry* in 1984. "The absence of body image on the wound image margins suggests that the blood images were present on the cloth before the body image was 'placed', 'appeared' or perhaps 'developed'." They further state, "Whatever the body-image production mechanism, it appears that it was prevented from acting by the presence of the blood/serum." If this concept is correct and if the body was not washed, then there would be patchy areas all over the Shroud showing an absence of the image because the image production mechanism would have been prevented by the presence of blood on the Shroud. Since there are no patchy areas showing an absence of body only images, then blood must have been absent in the image areas and the only way that blood would be absent from the Shroud is if *the body was washed.*

SCRIPTURE AND JEWISH BURIAL CUSTOMS

At the outset, it must be realized that my conclusion that the man of the Shroud was washed prior to placement on the shroud is made solely on a scientific basis. The following thoughts regarding scriptural support are presented with the full realization that I am not an expert in this area. However, my intention in presenting the following scriptural comments is merely an attempt to show that there is some scriptural support for the washing hypothesis. Ian Wilson's presumption (9) that many scriptural scholars believe Jesus was washed because they assume that the passage from St. John's Gospel "They took the body of Jesus and wrapped it with spices and in linen cloths following the Jewish burial customs" (John 19:40) is obviously correct because the passage is completely straightforward and clear in its interpretation. The evidence in favor of burial according to Jewish burial customs includes St. John's Gospel (John 19:40), The Lost Gospel According to Peter (section 6) indicated below, the strong probability of an object (shard) such as a coin over the eyes (see section on coins), the use of burial spices (John 19:39), and the wrapping in a shroud (19:40).

Rabbi Dan Cohn Sherbok of the University of Kent in England related that it was a legal obligation not only to enshroud the body but to wash and anoint it as well even on the Sabbath ("Jewish Shroud of Turin," Expository Times, 1981) However, Wilson's statement that "Only on the view that Jesus was not washed can the authenticity of the Shroud of Turin be upheld" basing it on the fact that there was not enough time to perform the washing since the Sabbath was at hand is completely untenable. A complete washing of the body accompanied by a shortened ritual can be accomplished in minutes. A piece of controversial scriptural evidence although not accepted by all religious scholars concerns The Lost Gospel According to Peter (section 6), which is hereby submitted because of its definitive statement regarding the fact that Jesus was washed prior to being placed on the shroud: "And he took the Lord and washed him, and rolled him in a linen cloth, and brought him to his own tomb, which was called the Garden of Joseph." This parchment codex was excavated in 1886 by the French Archaeological Mission when they excavated the grave of a monk in the Valley of the Upper Nile on the right bank of the river in the town of Akemin, which was called Panopolis. Historically, religious scholars recognized the existence of such a gospel. For example, reference to such a document was made in A.D. 190 by Serapion, Bishop of Antioch, in A.D. 253 by Origen, and in A.D. 300 by Eusebius, Bishop of Caesaria. In A.D. 455, Theodoret indicated in his Religious History that the Nazarines used The Gospel According to Peter. The "Stone of Unction," which had been recognized since the Byzantine era and was presently preserved in the Church of the Holy Sepulcher, is believed to be the stone on which Jesus was washed and anointed according to Wilson. Moreover, many scriptural scholars have opined the washing of the body prior to burial. Lavoie et al. present an excellent review of the Jewish law regarding burial customs through the sixteenth century. Although the major tenets of the law regarding burial customs at the time of Jesus were perhaps essentially the same as today, we do not know whether there are fine differences practiced today that were not practiced at the time of Christ's death. If we, however, must plug in some scientific justification for washing based on these modern practices, then I submit that the only blood flow after death included a small amount of a watery, blood-tinged discharge extruding from the lance wound. The amount of watery discharge and blood exuding from this wound had to be small because immediately upon the introduction of the spear into the chest cavity, the lungs would have collapsed due to the increased atmospheric pressure. Then the fluid level would have immediately dropped because there would have been more space in the chest cavity. Therefore, the only fluid extruding out of the wound would be from the initial penetration by the lance (immediately prior to collapse) and the small amount of blood from the right atrium of the heart contained on the spear tip by a quick, jerking motion following the sudden thrust. In my opinion, this amount is significantly less than the *quarter log* quantitated as the minimum amount of blood after death required to become unclean according to the Mishna and Talmud. All other blood on the body prior to washing would have been present prior to death and thus could be washed according to the Jewish prescription. If a rapid burial ceremony was necessary, the washing ritual could be effected and the body washed within a few minutes. Even if more than a quarter log extruded from the lance wound, the small amount of blood around the spear wound could have easily been avoided during the washing procedure. The act of washing would have then caused an oozing from each of the wounds thereby accounting for imprints consistent with those on the Shroud. The blood from these wounds could not have been subsequently washed because it would have been considered *unclean* blood. This scenario conforms to the requirements of Jewish law, accounts for the well-defined wounds depicted on the Shroud of Turin, and provides satisfactory explanation for the forensic pathologist.

IMAGE OF THE CRUCIFIED

The image of the body on the Shroud has characteristics that are in need of scientific explanation. The front of the neck appears to be absent, the legs and feet appear contradictory and the body appears somewhat asymmetrical. The explanation for the apparent absence of the neck is that the head is obviously bent forward in rigor motris. ["Then Jesus, crying with a loud voice, said, 'Father, into thy hands I commit my spirit!' And having said this he breathed his last" (Luke 23:46).] It was after these words that his head dropped forward in death, and the violence of his death caused a state of cadaveric spasm, or immediate rigor, as discussed previously, where the muscles of the neck contracted solidly, keeping the head bent forward until full rigor mortis set in.

Likewise, the legs, which were in a slightly bent position, with one foot almost flush to the cross, would maintain the same type of cadaveric spasm and subsequent rigor mortis prior to being taken down from the cross. The difference in height of the front image from that of the back image, with the latter being longer, supports this hypothesis of rigor mortis. Lorenzo Ferri, the eminent sculptor and sindonologist, measures a difference of 7 centimeters between the front and back images on a life-size reproduction of the Shroud.

HEIGHT OF THE CRUCIFIED

Precise measurements of the height of the crucified on the Shroud is fraught with difficulty because we are not dealing with an impression on a flat, rigid backing but a long length of cloth that was intricately tucked and folded over the crucified individual. In addition, there are other factors hindering preciseness such as the presence of rigor mortis, the effects of burial spices, the effects of weather conditions (sun, wind, and rain) during expositions, the unavailability of information as to whether the Shroud was on a sort of hard surface prior to placement of the body, how taut the Shroud was at the time of placement, and a multiplicity of other factors.

The height of the crucified has been estimated to be between 70.5 and 74 inches by various experts who directly measured the body image on the Shroud or measured the image from alleged full-size reproductions. Lorenzo Ferri, for example, reported that the body image was 186 centimeters (seventh-four inches); Father Peter Weyland estimated the height to be seventy-one inches when he measured the French Commission enlargements. Father Weyland, however, found that his enlargement of the Shroud itself was only 13'11¼" long, revealing a 3¼" discrepancy; the actual Shroud measures 14'3" long. This would afford a height of about 72½", which is still 1½" shorter than Ferri's estimate. An anatomist, Dr. Luigi Gedda, arrived at a measurement of seventy-two inches during the private exposition of the Shroud at Montevergine in 1946. Both Dr. Giovanni Judica-Cordiglia and Dr. Paul Vignon estimated the height of the man on the Shroud to be seventy inches, while Dr. Robert Bucklin reported a height of seventy-one inches. Most researchers would agree that the crucified of the Shroud was at least seventy-two inches in height, plus or minus one inch. This range of approximately six feet concurs with the height of six feet (183 centimeters) afforded by the Measuring Cross of the Emperor Justinian, which is in the ambulatory of St. John Lateran, in Rome. In this regard, three capable and trustworthy men were sent to Jerusalem in the seventh century by Justinian to determine the height of Jesus. They purportedly measured the Shroud then constructed a cross from these measurements.

How does this height of six feet compare with the average man of that time? Estimates given by anthropologists indicate that heights of 5'2" to 5'4" were average. The Giv'at ha Mivtar excavations did reveal twelve male skeletons that averaged 5'4" in height. One individual, however, was six feet in height. Unquestionably, the estimated height for the body of the man in the Shroud would have been considered tall for that time.

THE CROWN OF THORNS

The images corresponding to the forehead that represent blood (Figure 3-3) reveal a backward "3" impression on the left forehead position, a bifurcated stream on the right forehead, which continues into the hair, and several individual images on the brow and in the hair. Several tortuous streams are noted in the hair on both sides. This pattern is consistent with wounds created by the crown of thorns, which was plaited into a cap rather than into a circlet. The tridimensional, computerized photographs by Tamburelli (which will be discussed later) vividly portray many of these features.

The backward "3" configuration on the forehead has been postulated to be due to deep furrows of the forehead, but this is highly speculative because these furrows would have to be very deep, and, even then, I doubt if they would cause such a result. The more plausible explanation is that, following the removal of the cap of thorns, dislodgment of the clots of dried blood caused blood to ooze out of the puncture wounds. If the body was being carried to the tomb, the movements of the body would easily account for the tortuous flow.

The hypothesis that punctures by the thorns of branches of the frontalis arteries, which supply the forehead region, are responsible for the "3" configuration is untenable because even branches of a tiny arteriole (microscopic-sized arterial blood vessels) would have caused a torrent of blood, not a tiny, almost insignificant rivulet, and would soak the entire face and neck and perhaps the body. The head is a highly vascular region, that is, it contains myriads of blood vessels with the surface area abounding primarily with small capillaries. Therefore, it is more logical to presume that small surface capillaries were injured. Moreover, from a forensic point of view, it would be more likely that the postmortem dislodgment of the clots when removing the crown of thorns would cause a brief flow of blood down the forehead during movements of the body from the cross to the Shroud, with subsequent flows to the back of the head causing the pooling patterns of multistreams from the weight of the head against the Shroud.

The Shroud suggests excoriations and swelling of the forehead and of the brow, a bruise or swelling of the right upper lip, and swelling of the jaw. These observations are verified by the computer photos of Tamburelli (Figure 12-17), which will be discussed in this chapter under Tridimensional Analysis of the Turin Shroud.

BLOOD ON THE HAIR

The blood images depicted in the region of the hair on the frontal image of the Shroud has always been interpreted by just that—"blood on the hair" and never anything else. Recently, however, the Lavoies and Adler very ingeniously demonstrated that this may not be so; the blood may be on the face, not the hair. They made tracings on cloth of the blood wound images from a full-size negative image of the Shroud of Turin and made cutouts of the marks. They draped the cloth over the head of a bearded man so that the blood marks aligned with the man's face. They then applied paint through the cutouts. The blood marks all appeared on the face and not on the hair of the bearded man. They concluded that the blood images were a consequence of a contact with the front and sides of the face and independent of the body only image, giving an erroneous impression that the blood was in the hair. Unfortunately, however, this does not necessarily prove their point, but it does allow another possibility to explain these images. But the Lavoies and Adler's conclusions about image formation could only be valid if their results are definitively the only possibility. I also take exception with another one of their conclusions—that their study supports death while in the vertical position. Although I am convinced that death occurred while in the vertical position, I am not convinced that their study affords supporting evidence for this.

HANDS AND ARMS

It is not entirely correct to state that the imprint on the back of the left hand is over the wrist area. The wound in the region behind the palm is where the wrist meets the metacarpal bones of the back of the hand (Figures 8-2 and 12-13). This is portrayed in the tridimensional photograph by Tamburelli (Figure 12-18), which shows the fingers, back of the hand, wrist, and wound image in tridimensional relief. When a nail is driven through the thenar fissure of the palm, as indicated previously, the nail exits between the base of the metacarpal bones of the index and second fingers and the two corresponding carpal bones at a point corresponding to the imprint on the Turin Shroud.

It was demonstrated in a previous chapter that the bifurcation pattern is not due to the two hypothetical positions that the victim assumed on the cross. Observations in the medical examiner's office revealed that when clots caused by injuries of various types (bullet wounds, stabbings, and punctures) are disturbed in this area, rivulets of blood may run to the two sides of the ulnar styloid protuberance (the bump on the little finger side of the back of the wrist). It is, therefore, postulated that when the nail was removed from Jesus' wrist, a clot or smudge of dried blood was disturbed, causing an oozing of the blood to flow to the ulnar styloid protuberance, causing a divergence of streams.

DRAWING IN OF THE THUMB

Barbet first propounded the theory that the thumbs are missing on the Shroud because the nail injured the median nerve during its route through the wrist. He indicated that the median nerve was severed either halfway or two-thirds of the way each time the nail was pounded through Destot's space and drew the thumb

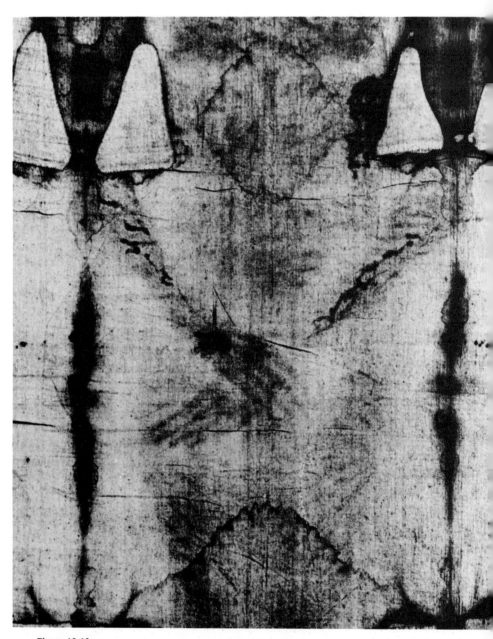

Figure 12-13

Shroud of Turin, lower chest and extremities.

This shows the bifurcation pattern on the hand (black and white arrows), wound on forearm (black arrows) and chest wound (white arrow).

into the palm. His explanation for this phenomenon is that the nail mechanically stimulates the median nerve when it severs it causing a contraction of the thenar eminence muscles with a drawing in of the thumbs. Not so! If the median nerve is damaged, it would momentarily *flex* and then *extend* (bend outward) and stay that way. This is confirmed by Dr. Ernest Lampe, one of the world's leading hand surgeons, who in discussing injuries to the median nerve in his book, *Surgical Anatomy of the Hand,* relates that in severance of the median nerve "There is inability to flex the thumb, index and middle fingers." I also consulted with several hand reconstruction surgeons and they all agreed that there might be an initial, rapid flexion followed by an extension. To explain Barbet's observation that the thumb bent sharply into the palm, I considered the possibility that perhaps when Barbet drove the square nail into the middle of the bending fold of the wrist, containing the transverse ligament, the nail may have compressed this ligament drawing the thumb into the palm, since two of the thenar eminence muscles are attached to the transverse ligament. I, however, had misgivings about this explanation when I observed that *the thumb of the cadaver that Barbet nailed to the cross was not flexed* (Figure 7-11).

There is, however, a very simple explanation why the thumbs are not visible on the Shroud. The thumbs are missing from the Shroud image because the natural position of the thumb, both in death and in the living person, is in the front of and slightly to the side of the index finger (see Figure 2-2 a and b). It would be next to impossible to have thumb impressions because the thumbs would never have even touched the Shroud. According to a 1980 article by Rhein in *Medical World News,* after hearing of my explanation, even Dr. Bucklin agreed that it might be so. He also said that some of the latest Shroud of Turin Research Project (STURP) (computer) photographs "show the thumb alongside the finger." In order to convince yourself, try the following: Place your hands to your sides and see where the thumbs are located relative to the rest of the hand. You will readily note that they are located in front of and slightly to the side of the index fingers. I have been expounding on this for many years, and I finally got through to a lot of Barbet devotees after the *Medical World News* article appeared. Every day deceased individuals are brought into the medical examiner's office, many of whom are transferred to our office from the local hospitals. These usually arrive with their wrists crossed and tied together. In

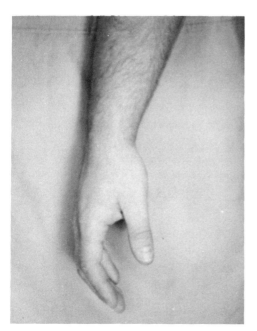 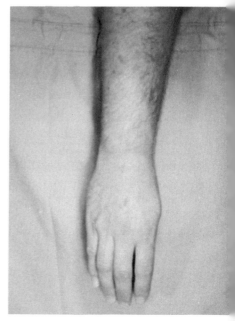

Figure 12-14
Position of the thumb.
Side (a) and back (b) of the hand. (a) The arm is naturally placed to the side with the palm facing the body. The thumb naturally resides in front of and slightly to the side of the index finger. Note that the thumb is not seen in (b).

every case, the thumbs are in a position in front of and slightly to the side of the index fingers.

ARM IMPRINTS

The imprints depicting the blood on the arms show a pattern of confluent streams almost to the elbow on the right side and an aggregate of rivulets directed in a diagonal direction toward the elbow and to the outside on the left arm. This has been interpreted by various sindonologists as resulting from the two positions assumed on the cross according to the asphyxiation theory, which was discussed previously and was found experimentally to be untenable. The most plausible explanation for these markings relates to the various positions assumed while the victim was removed from the cross and the arms lowered after dislodging clots of dried blood, thereby causing an oozing of the fluid of blood. A case that was investigated in the medical examiner's office is similar in principle. A young man who died as a consequence of multiple stab wounds to the chest also had a small stab wound of the wrist, which obviously occurred while defending himself. I examined the wound lightly with a small blood vessel probe at the scene. The blood appeared to be clotted or dried and was disturbed by the examina-tion. Subsequently, during the movement of the individual down the stairs to the morgue stretcher, with movements of his arms in the process, several streams of blood appeared down his arm in different directions. This type of liquid oozing would account for the imprints of the arm on the Shroud as indicated above.

SCOURGING

The imprints on the Shroud representing scourge marks are well defined, appear dumbbell-shaped for the most part, and are located over the back, shoulders, legs, chest, and abdomen (Figures 2-3 and 12-15). The counts vary from 100 to 120 impressions. It is of interest that two scientists, Lorre and Lynn, from the Pasadena Jet Propulsion Laboratory, analyzed scourge marks by creating a type of relief gradient using their IBM 360/65. This suggested that there were two directions, suggesting two different Roman soldiers on opposite sides of the victim (or one soldier changing to the opposite side). Since the scourge punctures would have been clot-ted prior to death, what would have been responsible for their impressing the Shroud? The well-defined borders of the scourge impressions make it evident that the body was washed prior to being placed on the Shroud; otherwise the impressions would be ill-defined (see section "the Man of the Shroud Was Washed After Death").

THE WOUND IN THE SIDE

After measuring the almost oval-shaped wound on the right side in life-size photographs, I am fully in agreement with the location reported by Dr. Barbet, which was between the fifth and sixth ribs, with the right side of the wound measuring about six inches from the center of the chest and the left lower side measur-ing a little over two and one-quarter inches from the center of the breastplate. A blood smudge below the oval wound area indicates that shortly after the spear thrust, some blood ran down the side of

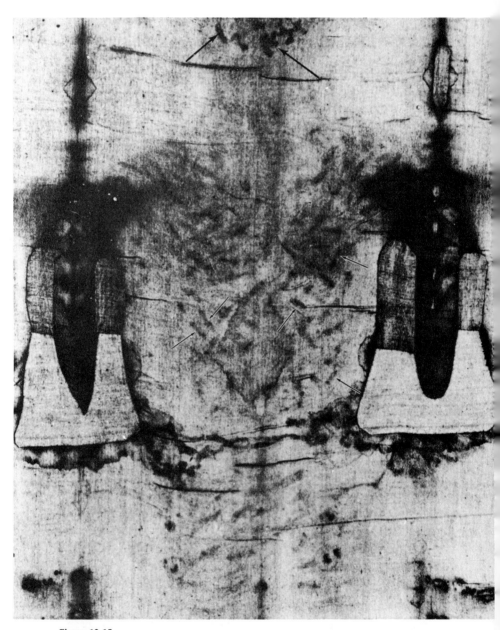

Figure 12-15

Shroud of Turin, blowup of back and back of the head.
The scourging pattern is depicted by the more than 100 dumbbell-shaped lash marks (black and white arrows). The pattern of these marks suggests that the soldier either changed position during the flogging or a second soldier alternated blows. Blood streamlets from the crown of thorns are also depicted (black arrows).

the chest, drying and clotting. Then, when the victim was re-moved from the cross and placed on the Shroud, some of the liquefied blood oozed out of the large wound to the back, causing the horizontal streams (Figure 12-15). The tridimensional pho-tographs of the Shroud by Tamburelli show suitable saturation of the chest wound (Figure 12-17). The amount of blood and watery discharge had to be small, i.e., less than a quarter log (see section "Jesus Was Washed").

FEET

An area of controversy resides in the interpretation of the image of the legs and feet. It is difficult to understand the presence of concomitant images of the back of the thighs, front of the thighs, the calves, the upper aspects of the front of the lower legs, and the entire sole of the foot, and the absence of an image in the front, lower aspects of the legs (Figure 12-30). Certainly, if the knees were bent in rigor mortis, even slightly so that the soles of feet were flush to the Shroud, neither the back of the thighs or knees would leave an image. How then, could one explain this image effect? One logical explanation is that when the body in rigor mortis was placed on the Shroud, the rigor in the knees was broken so that the legs would lay essentially flat. The excess cloth on the back of the body in the region of the feet was then drawn upward over the soles and around the toes to the top of the feet. Next, the cloth on the top of the body was drawn over the thighs, knees, and upper aspects of the lower legs directly to and then over the cloth of the toes. This explanation appears to be in accord with that of Fr. Werner Bulst, S.J.

The reason why there is no image of the sole of the right foot (except for a segment of the heel) and lower part of the left calf perhaps derives from either a very slight bending of the knee causing the foot to be slightly flexed forward, or the drawing inward of the left foot over the top of the right foot just above the toes of the latter. In the first instance, when the cloth was drawn up over the soles, it would have been flushed to the right sole but slightly away from the sole of the left foot, and in the second instance, the sole of the left foot would have been shielded from the cloth by the right foot. *It is important to note that both instances would explain the apparent shortening of the left leg.*

WAS JESUS ALIVE UNDER THE SHROUD?

Because Reban and others have indicated that Jesus was alive when he was placed under the Shroud, it seems necessary to dismiss this ridiculous concept. First, the Shroud shows strong evidence of rigor mortis (see section on rigor mortis). Second, if Jesus was alive under the cloth, the Shroud would have been literally saturated with blood from the numerous lacerations and wounds because even tiny wounds bleed profusely when the heart is beating. Third, if the spear had penetrated the chest and did not strike the heart, a pneumothorax (collapse of the lung) would occur because the pressure outside the chest is greater than within the chest, causing the lung to collapse. The other lung then becomes more inflated causing a shift of the heart structures that may result in cardiac arrest. Following the spear thrust, a sucking sound would have been obvious to the centurion and to the individuals who took Jesus down from the cross if he were alive. I responded to a call to the home of an individual who had been stabbed in the chest during a domestic dispute. The man was unconscious, but the sucking sound made by air being drawn into the chest through the blood and other body fluids could be heard across the room. Lack of reports of a sucking sound would be a direct refutation of the theory that Christ was alive after being taken down from the cross. And fourth, Pilate specifically checked with the centurion to be sure Jesus was dead before releasing the body to Joseph of Arimathea (Mark 15:43–45).

TRIDIMENSIONAL STUDIES OF THE SHROUD

TRANSFLEX METHOD OF VALA

The first tridimensional approach to the Shroud of Turin was done by Leo Vala, photographer, using his Transflex process of front projection. Two positives using the 1931 Shroud head photographs of Enrie were projected onto a bed of clay using two projectors (epidiascope) to provide the matrix for the bust. He was then able to sculpt the head, resulting in a full face image with plenty of gradational information. The basis of Vala's process as described by him relates to his concept that

> photographers, as a result of their unique type of training, see pictures differently from other people, but when you try to communicate what you

are feeling about vision to other people this is quite impossible, like trying to explain to a blind man what colour is—we do not have words for it. . . . Therefore, without realizing it the photographer looks at a full face picture and knows instinctively the shape of the man's nose, the shape of his cheeks, whether he has a weak chin or a weak forehead—he is seeing instinctively and without realizing it in three dimensions. Consequently, since we are trained to take a solid object and take it down into flat, then if we had a vehicle for it we could take a flat object and commit back into solid. This is the basis of my process which is very simple. ("The Turin Shroud," by Crawley.)

The result of Vala's experiment was impressive. He successfully created a three-dimensional representation of the head of the Shroud from a two-dimensional photograph.

COMPUTER IMAGING TECHNIQUE

Professor Paul Vignon, in the early part of this century during experiments with his vaporgraphic theory, noted that the image on the cloth varied inversely with the cloth to body distance. This observation set the stage for the three-dimensional computer imaging studies of Captains John P. Jackson, physicist, and Eric Jumper, of the United States Air Force Academy, and, later, Professor Giovanni Tamburelli from the University of Turin and director of research of the Centro Studi e Laboratori Telecomunicazione in Turin.

Jackson and Jumper in their experiments measured cloth to body distance, measured image intensity, and compared the cloth to body distance with the image intensity in different locations on the Shroud. The first aim was accomplished using a volunteer of a height similar to that of the image, whom they draped meticulously with a cloth onto which they projected a photo of the Shroud so that all image features lined up appropriately. They then took photos with and without the cloth in place so they could obtain body to cloth distances in a perpendicular plane from the ridge line (closest point of body to cloth). A microdensitometer was then used to follow the ridge lines to obtain a graphic record of the relationship of the image intensity of the body to cloth distance. They were able to conclude that Vignon's hypothesis was correct. They then subjected the image points of the Shroud photos to VP-8 image analysis as was previously done in processing Martian photographs three-dimensionally because the light source was at a distance. They obtained dazzling, tridimensional photos of the Shroud image, which they indicate is not possible with regular photography because the latter would show distortion with flattening of the relief including the arm within the chest and nose pressed into face. They also observed that, because the image produced no directional brush stroke marks such as might have been effected by an artist, forgery did not appear possible.

J. Germain of the United States Air Force Weapons Laboratory pointed out in the *Proceedings of the United States Conference of Research on the Shroud of Turin* in Colorado Springs that there was an error regarding the construction of the three-dimensional image and indicated that the adjustment of the gain to enhance certain areas such as the fainter portions of the image causes the head to grow out of proportion and if the gain is adjusted to develop a realistic nose, the fainter portions of the image are thrown completely or incompletely out of relief.

Professor Giovanni Tamburelli points out that the computer has the ability to channel the brilliance of the points in the photograph into corresponding numbers. He relates that in this way he can eliminate imperfections, lines, and spots, restore images in parts that appear out of focus or incomplete, and enhance images

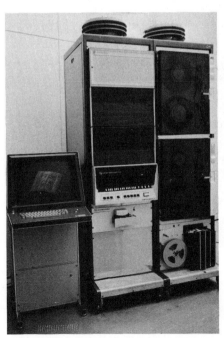

Figure 12-16
3-D imaging processing equipment.
Varian 620/i. Minicomputer (16 K Memory words) and a Tektronic videographic display.
(Courtesy of Prof. Tamburelli, CSELT, Turin, Italy).

by heightening details. Tamburelli used a Varian 620/i minicomputer (16K memory words) and a Tektronex videographic display (Figure 12-16).

TRIDIMENSIONAL EVALUATION
OF THE SHROUD

Head Region. A laceration appears to be present on the right cheek, across the nose, and on the left cheek near the nose. These marks have been interpreted by Tamburelli as caused by a single blow. The right cheekbone appears swollen, and there appears to be an excoriation over the left cheekbone. The nose shows typical Semitic characteristics, and the right eye contains a buttonlike object in relief that resembles a coin. Early Jewish practices included the placement of coins or pottery fragments to seal the eyelids. Tamburelli indicates that this use of coins was uncommon during the early Christian age and disappeared during the second

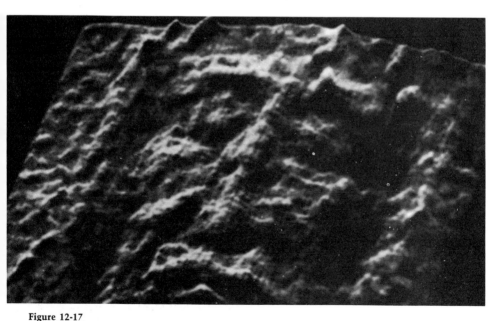

Figure 12-17
Shroud of Turin, 3-D relief of face.
A laceration is noted across the right cheek, nose and left cheek. Evidence of a coin-like object is seen in the right orbit of the eye. The blood flows on the forehead and hair stand out in sharp relief.
(Courtesy of Prof. Tamburelli, CSELT, Turin, Italy).

century, thereby adding another plus to the Shroud's authenticity (G. Ricciotte, *Vita De Gesu Christo* by Oscar Monadici, Sett., 1974).

The presumed blood patterns are vividly seen on the three-dimensional photographs (Figure 12-17). The tortuous flow noted on the left forehead on the Turin Shroud is strikingly shown in relief on the 3-D photos. Furthermore, the stream is now seen over the left eyelid, down the left cheek, and to the left lip, where it bifurcates into two small rivulets flowing into the beard. The two streamlets on the far right of the forehead are also pronounced. Tamburelli also interprets a flow on the right side of the nose, a clot at the lower right side of the lip, two streams of blood over the nostrils, a clot of blood in the central part of the upper lip, and a corresponding clot below that affords a well-defined character to the lower lip. The hair and beard appear to be "blood"-soaked.

Body Region. The tridimensional body image was processed by Tamburelli using a slight modification of the head technique (Figure 12-18). The fingers and hand stand out in sharp relief, and the saturation of the hand wound clearly reveals that the wound is indeed in back of the hand at a point where the wrist joins the metacarpal region of the back of the palm, as previously mentioned. The wound on the right side attributed to the spear wound has been suitably saturated, defining its position.

The Natural Face—Image Restoration and Enhancement. Tamburelli obtained remarkable 3-D reliefs of the face of the Shroud using recursive filters that eliminated the small wounds of the face and partially altered the larger wounds with elimination of the wound of the nose, smoothing of the forehead, and defining the eyelids and eyebrows. The results were outstanding and afforded a majestic appearance Tamburelli considers the "probable photograph of Jesus Christ" (Figure 12-19). He further points out that if the man of the Shroud was old and had wrinkles, they would be enhanced—which they are not—therefore providing evidence that the individual of the Shroud was relatively young.

The computer studies confirm the three-dimensional origin of the Shroud image, define the wounds and "blood" more clearly, reveal the location of the wound marks more precisely, reveal the possibility of coins over the eyes, and allegedly eliminate the

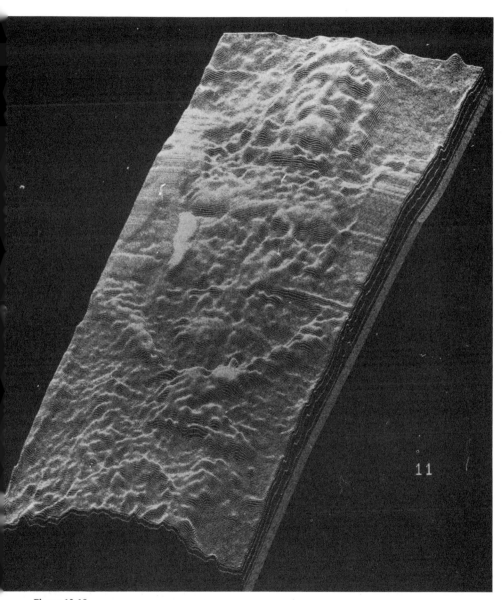

Figure 12-18
Shroud of Turin, 3-D relief of body.
Note that the hands are in sharp relief and the wound is behind the hand at a point between the wrist and metacarpal area. The wound on the right side stands out in stark relief.
(Courtesy of Prof. Tamburelli, CSELT, Turin, Italy).

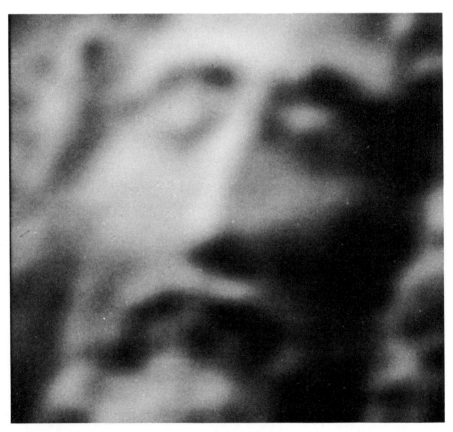

Figure 12-19
Shroud of Turin, 3-D relief of face.
Taken after smoothing out the rough transitions with a recursive filter.
(Courtesy of Professor Tamburelli, CSELT, Turin, Italy).

possibility that the man was old. Through image restoration, imperfection elimination, and image enhancement, a beautiful, probable photograph of the man of the Shroud results.

THEORIES OF IMAGE FORMATION

The mechanism by which an image was produced on the Shroud has remained a conundrum. It was hoped that the studies performed on the Shroud by the scientists following the 1978 exposition would finally put all doubts to rest and fully elaborate how the image was produced. Unfortunately, although much information was gleaned from these studies about the nature of the image, the mechanism has still evaded explanation leading to increased speculation and controversy.

Various proposed theories include the artistic or made by human artifice theory, the vaporographic theory of Vignon, the contact theory, the Volckringer theory, the photographic process theory, the scorch theory, the electromagnetic theory, the x-ray theory, and the hyperthermia-sodium carbonate theory.

ARTISTIC OR MADE BY HUMAN ARTIFICE THEORY

Historical Background. The question of an artistic forgery first arose in 1359, when Henry de Poitier, Bishop of Troyes, allegedly stopped Jean de Vergy, widow of Geoffrey de Charny from exhibiting the Shroud from which she was apparently profiting. Bishop de Poitier allegedly charged that the Shroud was fraudulent and that he had found the artist who had painted it. The Shroud was purportedly laid to rest for about thirty-two years until the de Charnys were quietly granted permission, with certain reservations, from anti-Pope Clement II to again exhibit it. The viewers had to be informed that the cloth was not the true burial cloth but a likeness or representation of the true Shroud. This reservation was supposedly met, but when the showing was discovered by Pierre d'Arcis—the new Bishop of Troyes—he allegedly sent a memorandum to Clement II, informing the Pope that some thirty years before, d'Arcis's predecessor, Bishop de Poitier, had discovered the fraud and found the artist who had cunningly painted it. Pope Clement II, however, purportedly silenced the Bishop, and allowed the de Charny family to continue with their exposition.

Since the time of the late nineteenth century historian, Ulysses Chevalier, the d'Arcis Memorandum has been the main fuel in maintaining the artistic theory. However, Rex Moran, editor of *Shroud News*, indicates the facts may be distorted. He wrote . . .

> research since the report by Chevalier early this century throws considerable doubt on whether the d'Arcis document was any more than an unsigned, undated and unsent memorandum, not even written by the said Bishop. There are several authentic papal documents concerning the exhibition of the cloth at Lirey, in France in the 1300s which reveal a dispute between d'Arcis and his predecessor and its then owners, the de

Charny family and there is authoritative and well researched current opinion that the d'Arcis document represents no more than a hasty judgement jotted down during the heat of a debate. (*Shroud News*, August, no. 30 1985)

In 1898, following Pia's photographic revelation, there was a surge of renewed interest in the Shroud by the scientific community. In the same year, however, the eminent historian Ulysses Chevalier, brought up old wounds by championing the forgery theory. He alleged that the image was painted in the fourteenth century and supported his charges with the old D'Arcis documents. A few years later, the noted Jesuit priest and scholarly writer, Herbert Thurston, wrote prodigiously against the authenticity of the Shroud; his arguments appeared for over fifty years in the *Catholic Encyclopedia,* the reference source for millions of Catholics. This was finally rectified by an excellent article submitted by Father Otterbein, a Redemptorist priest, which replaced Thurston's article on the Shroud.

Many attempts in the ensuing years to duplicate the image by paints, pigments, and stains have proved dismal failures because they lacked the fine, exacting gradations that made possible the inverted negative effect when tested photographically.

Photography. It is important to note at the outset that the concept of photography was unknown at the time of the de Charny-D'Arcis controversy since it was not invented until about 1822 when Jean Nicephore Niepce produced the first photographic image of the Shroud and called it heliography. Sir John Herschel changed the name to photography in 1839. Although Louis-Jacques Daguerre joined forces with Niepce and improved on the process somewhat, it was not until many years later that it was perfected. If an artist was perpetrating a fraud in 1359, how would he know what a photographic image was and furthermore what would he gain by producing a perfect photographic negative?

Enter McCrone. Walter C. McCrone, a formidable proponent of the artistic theory, is an internationally recognized microscopist and the director of the famous McCrone Associates Research Laboratory in Chicago. McCrone is well known for determining that the Yale University Vineland map was a forgery because it contained anastase, a titanium oxide material that had not been developed until about 1917.

After studying thirty-two sticky tape samples from various areas of the Shroud by using polarized light microscopy, scanning electron microscopy, energy dispersive x-ray analysis, electron microprobe analyzer, x-ray diffraction, and selected area electron diffraction, McCrone reported that the Shroud image was due to the application of red artists' pigment, which was intentionally added either to create the image or to enhance an earlier image. He further indicated that along with the red iron oxide, also known as red ochre, or Venetian red (an earth color), he found mercuric sulfide, another earth color known as vermillion, and a collagen tempra paint medium—all three of which have been used by artists throughout the centuries. McCrone also does not believe that the blood images are blood but believes the difference of color between the blood images and the body image relates to the amount of pigment present. In support of this he said that he got negative results for blood on the same samples for which Adler and Heller and Bollone independently reported positive results. He stated in his final conclusion in the *Skeptical Inquirer* (Spring, 1982):

> I can see no possible mechanism by which the shroud image could have been produced except as the work of an artist. The faithful representation of all of the anatomical and pathological markings, so well described in the New Testament would be difficult to produce except by an artist. They are totally without distortion and indeed look exactly the way we would like to have them look.

Comments. Before evaluating McCrone's iron oxide painting theory, it is necessary to review some of the most frequently used terminology and a few points of basic information. The *body only image* refers to the entire image excluding the areas of *blood stain images*. In this regard the body only image is entirely absent on the back of the Shroud but the blood stain images show completely through the cloth. The body only images are only present on the very top surface of the fibers with a penetration of only about two to three fibrils deep. The darkness of the body image appears to be determined by the number of fibrils in a unit area; the more fibrils present, the darker the image. The closer a person is to the image, the more difficult it is to see, and it literally fades away when one views it up close. Magnification of the image also makes it fade away making it very difficult to visualize.

Arguments against the *artistic theory*, including *McCrone's hypothesis*, primarily relate to the following:

1. It has been reported that there is no evidence of paintbrush marks as determined microscopically. Fourier analysis (a form of mathematical analysis of vibration patterns) showed no directionality. Lorre and Lynn analyzed the back image with IBM 360/65 and reported a purely random, unexplainable distribution of straight line forms with no directionality.
2. During pollen studies, Dr. Max Frei found that none of the pollens were glued to the cloth or covered with tempera thereby adding strong evidence against the Shroud being a painted fake.
3. Traces of paint pigments used by artists such as vermillion, etc. found by McCrone have been confirmed by other investigators. This is unquestionably understandable since many shrouds have been copied by artists directly from the Shroud of Turin. This is a relatively laborious process that involves grinding and mixing their paints in the same room containing the Shroud. Gusts of air and body movements could easily carry the pigment to the Shroud. Even more striking are the recent studies by Fossati of several famous shrouds actually laid flat upon the Shroud of Turin for some time in order to be recognized as a venerable relic. In particular the shrouds from the Spanish churches of Guadalupe and Navarette in 1568, Torres de la Alameda in 1620, La Cuesta in 1654, and Aglie in 1822 and in the United States, Our Lady of the Rosary (Summit, New Jersey) in 1624 were all laid flat, image to image, on the Shroud of Turin.
4. Following a comprehensive examination of the various stains and images on the Shroud, Jumper, Adler, Jackson, Pellicori, Heller, and Druzik in *Archaeological Chemistry III* (1984) reported the following:

   a. The fibrils in the body only image areas were determined to be yellow. This image is only visible because the superficial fibrils are more yellow than the nonimage areas.
   b. The cause of the yellow color that comprises the body only image is consistent with an aging effect due to an alteration of the microfibrils of the cellulose structure of linen caused by oxidation, dehydration, and conjugation of long chain sugar molecules comprising the microfibrils. The chromophore (chemical group that gives rise to color) appears to contain some type of conjugated carbonyl groups. When linen ages, it yellows at a slow rate due to decomposition. Something has caused an accelerated aging or advanced

decomposition effect in the body only image as compared to the surrounding nonimage areas. Deeper colored areas of the body only image merely reflects more of the yellowed fibers per surface area.

c. Experiments effected by Pellicori to accelerate the aging or decomposition process by controlled baking, with and without the application of foreign substances to the linen, such as perspiration, olive oil, etc., resulted in the reproduction of the same yellow coloration and spectral characteristics similar to those obtained on the Shroud. The application of heat apparently accelerates the decomposition process. In other words, what would have normally developed over a relatively long period is accelerated by heat in a matter of hours.

d. The color of the fibrils was subjected to solubility testing in organic solvents that covered the entire range of solubility and was found to be non-extractable. Strong acids or bases did not affect the color.

e. Since most of the organic dyes are affected by high temperatures, there should be some color changes in the image at the border of the scorch marks, which resulted from the fire of Chambéry, if such organic dyes caused the image. No such change is present. Since the silver casket containing the Shroud melted, the fire had to be very hot, an estimated 800 degrees centigrade. Since the body only image shows nonfluorescence, many organic dyes can be eliminated.

f. The color on the fibrils does not arise from inorganic pigments. Moreover, there is no correspondence of the body only images to the concentration of iron oxide since the spectral characteristics of the body only image are different from those of iron oxide. The color of the fibers, due to iron oxide, is also precluded by the fact that oxidation or reduction converts the yellow fibrils of the body only image to a white color. Only occasional particles of iron oxide are noted on the body only image fibrils. Large amounts of iron bound to the cellulose of the Shroud (not iron oxide) and calcium were both present throughout the Shroud. This is believed to be due to the ability of linen to bind iron and water by ion association during the retting process in the manufacture of linen from flax when the linen was immersed in water during fermentation. An estimated 90 percent exists in this bound form to the cellulose of the linen and only a small amount is present as iron oxide. These iron oxide components probably arise from the conversion of some of the iron in the margins of the water stains to mineral khaki. Similar tests on samples taken from a 300 year-old piece of Spanish linen, from a Coptic Funerary linen dating to about A.D. 350, and a Pharaonic linen dating to about B.C. 1500 all gave similar results for calcium and iron.

g. All of the iron examined from the Shroud, whether from iron oxide particles or from blood, proved to be about 99 percent chemically pure with no manganese, nickel, or cobalt discernable. The earth pigment, red ochre, (Venetian red) from either medieval or older sources used abroad were contaminated with manganese, nickel, or cobalt greater than 1 percent.

h. X-ray studies of the body only image do not contain enough iron oxide to show up on the x-radiographs (opinion of McCrone). If natural water soluble dyes were present they would have migrated when the water stain markings occurred. This did not appear to have occurred.

i. The body only image areas do not fluoresce under ultraviolet light while the scorch areas do in the areas of the blackened fibers. This was determined due to the formation of pyrolytic products with combustion in a reduced oxygen atmosphere.

j. Testing with microchemical tests, laser microprobe Raman spectroscopy, and mass spectroscopy failed to reveal evidence of added materials on the fibrils of the body only image fibrils.

k. There is no evidence of any cementing between fibrils in the body only image areas. Moreover, the fibrils in this area gave negative results when tested for protein down to a thousandth of a milligram, using sensitive tests including the fluorescamine method, protease digestion, and the amido black test. The amido black test, if used alone and without controls as McCrone did, however, may give misleading results becuase it may also stain oxidized cellulose.

l. The blood images were clearly blood and likely of human origin with nothing else present that would be suspect. There was no evidence of an artistic enhancement of a preexisting blood image or that the blood images were painted.

m. In the blood image areas, the fibrils appear cemented together. These fibrils gave a positive test for protein. This was also reported by Schwalbe and Rogers and by Pellicori. The latter also noted that there was a coating of the fibers and variegation of color. All in all, the color in the blood image areas appeared different than in the body only image areas.

n. In conclusion, these investigators indicate that they do not have a satisfactory, simple explanation for how the image got on the cloth, and they found it highly improbable that the image was artistically produced.

THE RUBBINGS OF JOE NICKELL

In 1978, Joe Nickell, whose scientific and medical expertise includes teaching technical writing, performing as a magician and working as a detective agency investigator, published in the *Humanist* (November/December, 1978) and in *Popular Photography* (November 1979) a rather interesting rubbing technique to create images in positive and negative from bas reliefs of Bing Crosby. He soaked cloth in hot water and molded it to contours of the relief with a blunt tool, then allowed it to dry. He then made a powdered mixture consisting of equal parts of myrrh and aloes and carefully applied the powder with a cotton dauber. Later, he performed the same technique using iron oxide, as per McCrone's finding, and was able to prepare similar but more intense images. Recently, Nickell has allegedly changed his approach somewhat and is entertaining the hypothesis that the iron oxide (ferric oxide with traces of ferrous oxide) in his rubbing technique produced the image by causing a degradation of the cellulose fibrils. Through the years, most of the iron oxide would fall off, leaving only some remnants of the iron oxide pigment.

COMMENT

At the outset, it must be realized that the ability to produce an image in the negative and positive does not prove that the image was produced by an artist and that the Shroud is a fraud. Even McCrone, who believes that the Shroud was the product of an artist, did not make wild accusations that the Shroud is a fraud as Nickell alleges, but indicated that he felt an artist was "commissioned to paint a shroud." McCrone has probably worked on enough forensic cases to understand that the D'Arcis memorandum provided no proof for the accusations as to who the artist was, if there really was one, or the circumstances surrounding the alleged confession. Nickell's unscientific approach in his book, *The Inquest,* is reminiscent of the approach of individuals who pull things out of context in the Bible to prove their point or to build up the credentials of one person and avoid the excellent credentials of another person they wish to put down.

Nickell's work suffers from its failure to provide a finely detailed computer image, both in the negative and positive, comparable to that of the Shroud. Nickell's alleged new modification of his theory (discussed above) is also defective in that (1) studies show no differences in the iron oxide content in the body only image areas as compared to the off image areas, (2) the iron on the Shroud is 99 percent chemically pure with no discernable manganese, nickel, or cobalt. Red ochre, from either medieval or older sources, was contaminated with manganese, nickel, or cobalt greater than 1 percent and (3) the rubbing technique does not afford a cloth-body distance relationship when subjected to computer VP-8 image analysis. Purportedly, McCrone does not agree with Nickell's recent hypothesis believing that the iron oxide was applied by a brush and should be all over the fibrils. In contrast, when one examines the fibrils of one of Nickell's rubbings, the iron oxide is bunched up on one side of the fibrils. In order to place any credence in Nickell's hypothesis, one would have to subject it to rigorous testing. First of all, Nickell would have to produce a complete, duplicate, life-size image on a comparable piece of linen, both front and back with all of the fine details shown on the Shroud of Turin, including the scourge and other wound markings, arms crossed at the wrists, peculiar leg and foot images, etc. Next, the resultant "shroud" would have to be subjected to conditions simulating the Chambéry fire. Then, it would have to be analyzed with visible, infrared, and ultraviolet spectroscopy, x-ray fluorescence, x-radiographic imaging, infrared thermography, scanning electron microscopy, microchemical tests, etc., and give similar results. Next, sticky tape samples would have to be taken for a comprehensive chemical, biophysical, microscopic, scanning electron microscopic, x-ray, optical examination, etc., also with similar results. In addition, all the images and stains on the "shroud" would have to be similar. Lastly, computer image analysis would have to be performed to determine if a cloth-body distance relationship is presented. If the Shroud of Nickell didn't satisfy all of the criteria, it couldn't be accepted as a legitimate challenge to the authenticity of the Shroud of Turin.

THE VAPORGRAPHIC AND RELATED THEORIES

The first attempt to scientifically explain the Shroud images was made in 1902 by Professor Paul Vignon, a biologist from Paris. His findings were presented before the French Academy of Science by Professor Yves Delage, a well respected comparative anatomist and avowed agnostic from the prestigious Sorbonne. Unfortunately, his lecture was met with much resistance and marred his reputation among his colleagues.

After studying effects of paints and dyes on linen and direct contact of pigments, Vignon found a correlation between ammonia vapors given off by the body and the aloes used in the burial process. "And there also came Nicodemus, who at first had come to Jesus by night, bringing a mixture of myrrh and aloes, in weight about a hundred pounds. They therefore took the body of Jesus and wrapped it in linen cloths with the spices, after the Jewish manner of preparing for burial" (John 19:39–40). Vignon postulated that urea present in sweat and blood degrades, giving off ammonia vapors that rise from the corpse and react chemically with (oxidize) the aloes placed on the cloth, resulting in a brown coloration. He found that the image intensity varied inversely with the cloth to body distance. In other words, the farther the parts of the body were away from the cloth, the farther the ammonia vapors had to rise, resulting in a less intense image of that part and vice versa. Experiments were subsequently conducted by saturating statues and corpses with ammonia and soaking the linen in a mixture of oil and aloes. Negative images appeared on the linen cloth but never to the perfection of the Shroud. The *vaporgraphic hypothesis* of Vignon is no longer tenable for several reasons. First, the ammonia would diffuse into the cloth causing a blurred image unlike that of the Shroud. Second, the image would not be confined to the surface fibrils since the ammonia would diffuse into the cloth causing the image deep to the weave of the fibers. It has been shown that only the top most surface contains the body only image. And third, the color of the body only image on the Shroud is yellow while the images produced by Vignon are brownish.

THE CONTACT HYPOTHESIS

The contact approach was first attempted by Vignon prior to his developing the vaporgraphic hypothesis. He used ground up red chalk, which he applied to his facial area after wearing a fake moustache, and had assistants gently press a linen cloth containing albumin on his face. The resulting image was badly distorted, and Vignon abandoned this approach. He reasoned that, in concept, a contact hypothesis could not possibly produce an undistorted image of a face, which is very irregular and in different planes, because, when the image of the face was laid out flat, it would result in a distorted, larger impression. Following the Exposition of 1932, there was renewed interest in the contact hypothesis by two forensic medicine experts, Drs. Romanese and Judica-Cordiglia and a chemist, Dr. Scotti from Turin. Romanese soaked a cadaver with a salt solution resembling sweat then placed a linen cloth containing powdered aloes over the body and obtained negative images of the body. Dr. Judica-Cordiglia placed blood on the corpse, a linen cloth that had been soaked in a mixture of aloes, turpentine, and oil over the body, and hot steam. He succeeded in producing images with gradations that resulted in negative images but not approaching anything near the quality of the image on the Shroud. Later Professor Sebastiano Rodante of the International Center of Sindonology carried on experiments using the damp environment of the Catacombs where he sprayed the faces of corpses with Harnach's formula, consisting of two parts solution resembling sweat and one part blood. He also placed trickles of blood on the forehead that he allowed to dry. A linen cloth soaked in a watery mixture of aloes and myrrh was then placed over the face and allowed to lie for different periods of time resulting in negative images of the face with positive images of blood. The optimal time was about thirty-six hours, not incompatible with the time that Jesus lay in the tomb. But again the results were markedly inferior to the image on the Shroud.

Comment. *At the outset, one can definitively state that all of the contact hypotheses described above are now fully discounted because the intensive scientific examinations conducted following the 1978 Exposition ruled out aloes as causing the image,* since the body only image has been determined to be yellow in color while the images produced by the aloe-contact methods are brownish. Although we cannot fully discount a contact hypothesis, per se, there are various reasons why a contact mechanism could not adequately explain the body only images particularly in the head region, while it does, however, appear to explain the blood images. Even the best of the contact images of the head produced by the above techniques were markedly inferior to the image on the Shroud. For a contact hypothesis there are two major criticisms, however, regarding the body only images of the head region. The first relates to the distortions that occur with contact procedures. When the cloth is pressed on the front and sides of the face and then laid flat, a widened severely distorted image results. The second criticism relates to the inability of contact mechanisms to produce an appropriate cloth-body distance effect as has been demonstrated on the Shroud. The computer image enhancement studies appears to encode tridimensional information consistent with the Shroud being draped over a human body. Moreover, images appear to be present in areas where there would be no cloth-body contact.

The contact hypothesis does, however, appear to account for blood image areas such as the scourge marks and the fine scratches shown in the photo taken by Miller and Pellicori by the process of ultraviolet fluorescence photography in *Biological Photography* (Vol. 4, p. 78, 1981). It is interesting that in the ultraviolet photos of some blood wound images, particularly around the hand wound image (page 82 of the same article), there are clear areas devoid of image suggesting that perhaps the blood images were present before the body only image was produced. This would provide additional support for the hypothesis that the man of the Shroud was washed prior to placement on the Shroud (See section "The Man of the Shroud Was Washed After Death").

Pellicori's hypothesis discussed under the scorch hypothesis is in essence a contact mechanism based on the concept that burial ointments or natural body substances pass into the Shroud and in a sense catalyze or accelerate a cellulose degeneration in the areas containing these substances. The weakness of the hypothesis resides in the inability to account for the non-distorted facial image (Refer to scorch hypothesis).

VOLCKRINGER'S HYPOTHESIS

A very interesting hypothesis stems from the 1942 observations of Jean Volckringer, a pharmacist from St. Joseph's Hospital in Paris. Dr. Volckringer noted that certain plant herbs pressed in a book for many years frequently produce striking, finely detailed, images of the plants complete with venation patterns (Figure 12-20a) on the pages above and below the plant and sometimes projecting the image to an additional page below. He also noted that the herbs had to have been in the book a long time to produce an image because none of the recent herbs, even one that had been pressed in a book for thirty-four years, produced an image. However, another herb over a century old gave a very clear, well-defined

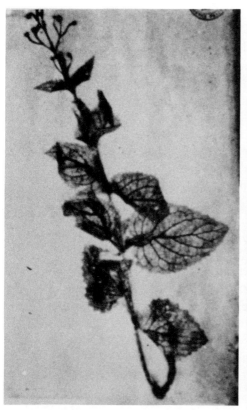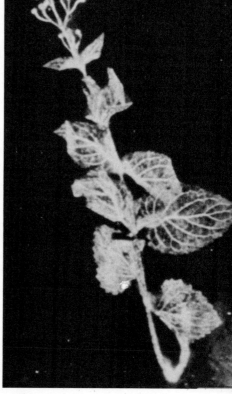

Figure 12-20
Negative and positive Volckringer patterns.
(a) As seen in a book.
(b) Appearance on a photographic negative.

image. When photographs of this image was taken, a positive image was produced on the negative film (Figure 12-20b) like that which occurs when the Shroud is photographed. Moreover, the coloration of the image is similar to the color of the body only image seen on the Shroud. There is, however, one essential difference, the image on the Shroud is only present on the surface of the fibrils while in the Volckringer patterns, the image penetrates into the paper. The Volckringer patterns have long held an esteemed place in Shroud studies, though primarily as a curiosity. In recent years, however, there has been renewed interest since recent studies indicate that the body only image may be a consequence of an accelerated decomposition of the cellulose fibrils in the area of the image. The book paper containing the Volckringer patterns

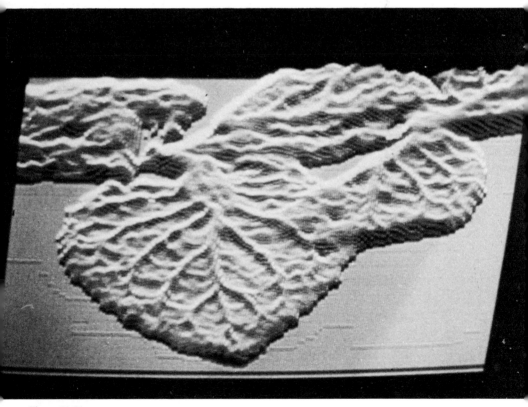

Figure 12-21
3-D relief of Volckringer pattern.
Reconstruction of leaf from Figure 12-20.
(Courtesy of Dr. John DeSalvo.)

also contains a high content of cellulose indicating a similar mechanism in the production of the image. In view of this, Dr. John DeSalvo, a biophysicist, decided to compare the visible spectral reflectance data of the Volckringer patterns with the data derived from the body only image of the Shroud obtained by the Gilberts in 1978. DeSalvo found almost identical patterns. He then checked the ultraviolet pattern and found an absence of fluorescence under ultraviolet light in the Volckringer patterns. He finally subjected the image to a VP-8 Image Analyzer and obtained an excellent 3-D relief (Figure 12-21).

It appears that acids from the plant, including lactic acid, are transferred to the paper, altering the cellulose structure at the sites of transfer over long periods of time. DeSalvo then hypothesized his revised vaporgraphic-direct contact hypothesis, which proposes two mechanisms to explain the image on the Shroud. The first is a direct contact mechanism in which the man in the Shroud would have large amounts of lactic acid on his skin from profuse sweating caused by torture and crucifixion that would transfer to the cloth to produce an image on the Shroud over a long period of time. DeSalvo speculated that the lactic acid would not penetrate the Shroud as it did on the book page on the Volckringer patterns because of low absorbency of the Shroud. The second mechanism is a molecular diffusion process to explain the three-dimensional nature of the image since the lactic acid concentration is greatest in areas of the cloth closest to the body, thereby causing the greatest degree of cellulose degradation and vice versa.

Comment. The Volckringer hypothesis has much merit because of the sharpness, clarity, and lack of distortion of the images, the similarity in color, the high cellulose content, the ability to produce a sharp, concise positive image on the negatives, and the tridimensionality of the image. There is little doubt from a forensic pathological evaluation that the man of the Shroud was washed prior to placement on the Shroud making the lactic acid hypothesis difficult to accept for the Shroud image. Moreoever, even if the lactic acid in sweat were present on the Shroud, it might account for an image in areas of contact but would not account for the cloth-body distance relationship noted on the Shroud despite DeSalvo's proposal. It is for the same reason that Pellicori's theory also based on his experiments in which skin secretions, simulated by the use of perspiration plus oils and olive oil, followed by controlled baking is not acceptable because both molecular transport systems require contact with the cloth for image production. Since the image is not present throughout the weave structure, a vapor diffusion does not appear acceptable. Since DeSalvo has not performed any experiments relating to his hypothesis, it is suggested that he test part of his hypothesis by allowing solutions simulating human sweat to evaporate onto linen samples over a thirty-six-hour period and then bake the linen under control conditions as Pellicori did to markedly accelerate the process. The sweat solution should be prepared according to the composition of sweat following intensive muscular activity since the lactic acid content would be markedly higher.

PHOTOGRAPHIC PROCESS THEORY

A very interesting concept was proposed by Geoffrey Crawley in an article in the *British Journal of Photography* on March 24, 1967:

> Apparently, it is an historic fact that the Shroud was kept in a silver casket for centuries and the burn marks sustained during the burning of the Chambéry Castle Chapel were caused by the melting of this silver casket in the heat. . . . Perhaps, as a result of a body lying in this Shroud, certain chemical materials or latent impressions were left in the fibers. Could some type of reaction have occurred during the centuries the Shroud lay in the silver casket? Did the heat of the burning castle then 'develop up' the impression? . . . Did some pious, artistic monk, overwhelmed by the miraculous appearance of this impression and realizing it showed no marks of crucifixion then set about adding the "positive" wound marks?

Recent studies, however, have demonstrated that only occasional, tiny specks of silver are present, and only in the scorch areas, thus completely negating the photographic process theory.

SCORCH RADIATION THEORIES

When I observed the Turin Shroud during the 1978 exposition, the scorch theory propounded by Geoffrey Asche in 1966 came to my mind because the coloration of the image reminded me of an ironing board cover that had been scorched. Asche heated a medallion of a brass horse in relief and gently pressed it against a handkerchief held taut. A scorched negative image of the horse resulted after a few seconds and the photographic negative showed an inversion of light values. Asche speculated that a brief and violent burst of some type of radiation other than heat scorched the Shroud during the resurrection, and he concluded as follows: "The acceptance of the Holy Shroud as a 'scorch picture' whatever the precise mode of creation, justifies the following statement; 'The Shroud is explicable if it once enwrapped a human body to which something extraordinary happened. It is not explicable otherwise.'"

The areas in which the Shroud was burned in the Chambéry fire are referred to as the scorch areas. The linen fibrils in these areas show different degrees of scorching from lightly scorched (light brown) to severely scorched (black). The scorch areas were found to fluoresce under ultraviolet light while the body image areas do not. Many people have abandoned the scorch theory because of this finding.

Comment. Studies have shown a striking similarity in both physical and chemical characteristics between the body image fibrils and the lightly scorched fibrils. Both have undergone an accelerated aging or decomposition process in the linen (dehydration, oxidation, and conjugation of multiple bonds in the cellulose molecular structure) but on the scorched fibrils the process was more rapid and destructive (see section under "Artistic theory, Comment"). In order for the scorch theory to be applicable, a more gentle thermal producing effect would have to be operative. It is interesting that Pellicori's experiments to accelerate the aging or decomposition process by controlled baking, with and without the application of foreign substances like perspiration and olive oil to the linen, reproduced the yellow coloration and spectral characteristics similar to those he had obtained on the Shroud. The application of heat merely accelerates the decomposition process. In other words, what would have normally developed over a relatively long period is accelerated by heat in a matter of hours. Pellicori's hypothesis suggests that perhaps burial ointments were transferred to the Shroud by contact and the ointments catalyzed cellulose degeneration in the areas of contact. The shortcomings of Pellicori's hypothesis derive from the fact that although it might go far in explaining the body image by contact, it does not explain the non-distorted facial image depicted on the Shroud (see section "contact hypothesis").

RADIATION MODIFICATION

A modification of the scorch theory relates to a brief *radiation* effect. Proponents of this modification hold that the image may have been formed by an intense, extremely brief (in milliseconds) burst of radiant energy. This is often referred to as a 'flash photolysis.' An analogy has been drawn between the Shroud image and the images formed on rocks, roads, and the sides of buildings in Hiroshima after the atom bomb blast. This is vividly described by John Hersey in his book *Hiroshima.* During the assessment of the bomb damage, Japanese scientists found that 'the flash of the bomb had discolored concrete to a reddish tint. . . . had *scorched* certain other types of building material . . . left prints of the shadows that had been cast by its light.' These included a permanent shadow on the roof of the chamber of commerce building of its rectangular tower, a shadow of a gas pump handle, several shadows cast on tombstones, and shadows of the parapets imprinted on the road surface of the Yorozuyo bridge (Figure 12-22). In one case, a human shadow was cast on the steps at the entrance to the Sumitomo Bank in Kamiyacho about 250 meters from the hypocenter (Figure 12-23). The stones containing the shadow are preserved at the Hiroshima A-Bomb Memorial Museum. Hersey relates that the above findings resulted in fanciful stories such as the findings of a shadow of a painter in the act of dipping his brush cast on the front of a bank and an embossed shadow of a man about to whip a horse cast on a bridge, but these have not been confirmed.

Comment. The source of the intense radiation, however, has evaded scientific explanation, and many devout Christians believe that it is of divine origin, representing the moment of resurrection. Since the artistic theory could not be confirmed and appears highly improbable because of an absence of dyes, stains, or pigments in sufficient quantity to cause an image, since no satisfactory explanation for the origin of the image on the cloth has been identified, and since the Shroud body only image appears to be related to a cloth-body distance relationship suggesting a projection mechanism of some unknown type, a thermal hypothesis of some type, capable of causing a gentle decomposition (accelerated aging effect) on linen cannot be ruled out.

Figure 12-22
Shadows of parapets.
Cast on road surface of Yurozuvo Bridge, Hiroshima. (Photos: U.S. Army.)

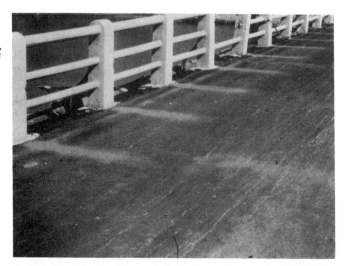

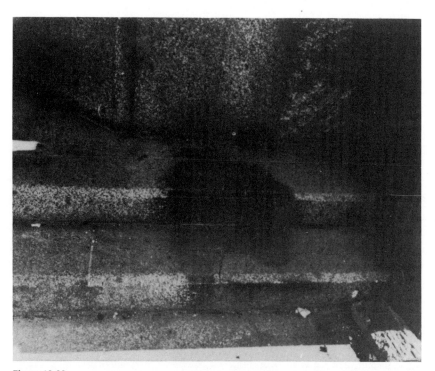

Figure 12-23
Shadow of human figure.
Cast on Sumitomo bank steps, Hiroshima. (Photo: U.S. Army.)

ELECTRICAL DISCHARGE MODIFICATION

Several investigators independently proposed that the image on the Shroud is due to a scorching effect from high voltage, high frequency electrical discharges. Dr. Scheuermann, a German physicist, has subjected linen to radiation from high voltage, high frequency discharges and has produced images showing many of the features of the images on the Shroud. Dr. Igor Benson, an engineer and Russian Orthodox priest from North Carolina, has also applied this concept to Shroud research but has focused on the role of ball lightning in producing the image. His theory, indicated in the September 1984 issue of *Shroud News*, is based on the hypothesis that when the man of the Shroud was lying in the tomb, a violent electrical storm might have occurred and ball lightning might have been the culprit by striking the body, charging it with high voltage energy that would almost immediately have dissipated its ionizing energy (discharge), thereby scorching the cloth and producing the image. Benson's experimental studies are conducted by directing a high energy source from a cathode energy tube located within a glass ball to a linen cloth.

In the June 1985 issue of *Shroud News*, Rex Morgan presented the hypothesis of Dr. Graeme Coote, a physicist from New Zealand, that suggests that during an earthquake, stresses on rock containing quartz crystals can generate high voltage. Considering this, Coote referred to the New Testament, which indicates that an earthquake occurred at about daybreak on the Sunday after the death of Jesus. "Now after the Sabbath, toward the dawn of the first day of the week Mary Magdalene and the other Mary went to see the sepulchre. And behold there was a great earthquake." Coote quotes in *Shroud News*:

> I am convinced that the image on the outside surfaces of the Shroud resulted from the bombardment of electrons and positive ions accelerated by an electrical field, which may have been present for a number of hours, causing a glow discharge. The field direction may have changed direction several times as the earthquake waves passed. Because the accelerated ions only have a short range in matter, the scorch would be very shallow, as observed. The properties of the electrostatic field containing the body (a conductor) and the Shroud (an insulator) lead naturally to the projective property of the image and the "photographic negative" property.

Comment. Although the electrical discharge hypotheses described above appear implausible, they must be fully tested since they are purported to give a projection mechanism, to effect a cloth-body distance mechanism, to code three-dimensional information, to present a negative image, and to show that the images affect the superficial aspects of the linen fibrils. Unfortunately, a good experimental model for testing these hypotheses does not yet exist.

X-RAY HYPOTHESIS

The x-ray hypothesis was proposed by Dr. Giles Carter, an archaeological chemist at Eastern Michigan University who subjected linen samples to x-rays and produced images with about the same coloration as that of the Shroud. According to Carter, x-rays appear to be a more plausible source than light rays because (he seems to think that) bones and teeth are visible in the image. Moreover, he also indicates that x-rays also cause the oxidation and dehydration or accelerated aging effect on linen as was hypothesized by scientists who investigated the Shroud after the 1978 Exposition. According to the x-ray hypothesis, the high energy rays would react with silicon and sodium in the dirt and salt on the skin surface and emit secondary, soft x-rays, which would produce the image. The variable intensity of the image would be due to the emission of x-rays from different skin levels and the fainter portions as a result of absorption of x-rays by the air between. X-ray emissions would also explain the cloth-body distance relationship, which, by using the VP-8 image analyzer, appear to give a three-dimensional effect of the Shroud image. He explains that the bones, seen in the image of the hands, were not formed directly by x-rays from bones because the x-rays would have been too energetic passing right through the fabric without a trace. Instead, according to Carter, the bone images are accounted for by the more intense images of the finger skin between the bone and cloth.

Comment. Alan Adler related that the x-ray hypothesis is "great physically, great chemically but absolutely bizarre biologically. Anyone who was that radioactive would be dead long before he was crucified" (*Chemical and Engineering News*, February 21, 1981), yet still, one must not totally disregard it. Since it appears sound scientifically, and if Carter is successful in producing a satisfactory image, then, like the thermal hypothesis, it cannot be totally ruled out.

HYPERTHERMIA-CALCIUM CARBONATE HYPOTHESIS

The hyperthermia-calcium carbonate hypothesis was proposed by Joseph Kohlbeck, an optical crystalographer with the Hercules Aerospace Division, and Eugenia Nitowski, an archaeologist, Carmelite nun, and expert in the archaeology of ancient tombs of the Israeli-Jordan region.

The finding of calcium carbonate on the Shroud fibers led them to ask whether the calcium carbonate originated from limestone in a first century Judean tomb. The first phase of their work was to determine the effects of a limestone-water paste on linen fibers. Kohlbeck and Nitowski reported a mercerization effect in which the slightly alkaline limestone attacked the outer skin of the fiber producing a yellow color they indicated was due to small amounts of iron in the limestone that was carried in the water to the fiber. Both agree that the image on the Shroud must be due to a change within the cellulose and not due to particles attached to the fibers. They then postulated that since heat speeds up the mercerization process, the key to image formation must derive from high temperatures generated in the form of a heat stroke from the effects of the hematidrosis, scourging, and crucifixion. An experimental model using a three foot tall medical manikin was filled with water that had been heated to a temperature between 110 and 115° Fahrenheit. They then wrapped the manikin in pure, untreated Belgian linen, which had been lightly dusted with calcium carbonate followed by the addition of an artificial "sweat" solution made by adding acetic acid to normal saline. The shrouded manikin was then placed in a totally dark basement having a temperature of 62 to 65° Fahrenheit and a relative humidity from 58 to 66 percent. A water mist was sprayed over the shrouded manikin and left for a period of thirty and one-half hours. They reported the production of an image in "areas of the manikin's body that retained heat the longest, namely the chest and back." According to this hypothesis, a high skin temperature resulting from heat stroke and acidic sweat in a humid environment accelerated a mercerization of the linen fibers, and the alkaline limestone (calcium carbonate), which had rubbed onto the shroud, caused a yellow image by virtue of the iron contained in the limestone.

Their hypothesis is untenable for several reasons. In the first place, the extensive crucifixion studies performed in my laboratory revealed that the crucified died of traumatic and hypovolemic shock that had begun with the hematidrosis and brutal scourging and increased in intensity with each subsequent event (such as the crowning with thorns, nailing of the feet and hands, the traumatic, postural and sweating effects on the cross, etc.). *One of the primary signs of shock is a reduction in skin temperature characterized by "cool, pale, moist skin."*

Secondly, the skin in *heat stroke* is *not* sweaty but extremely *dry and hot with an absence of sweating* because there is a dysfunction of the heat-regulating mechanism. The authors attempt to support their theory, a priori, by quoting from Barbet's book regarding observations made at the Dachau concentration camp; ". . . This sweat was especially abundant, indeed to an extraordinary extent, during the last few minutes before death . . ." and by quoting from my crucifixion studies where I indicated that a "marked sweating reaction became manifest in most individuals." This is entirely true but temperatures taken during the sweating episodes in my experiments were never hyperthermic and varied between 96 to 99° Fahrenheit on numerous volunteers. Neither of these quotes, however, support the hypothesis of *heat stroke* since this condition is manifested by "*high fevers* and *cessation of sweating* with dry skin."

It is important not to confuse *heat stroke* with the medical condition known as *heat exhaustion*, which is due to marked dehydration and is characterized by normal or slightly elevated temperatures, weakness, profuse sweating, and intense thirst. It is of interest that the features exhibited during the crucifixion appear to fit more appropriately into *heat exhaustion*. The feature of thirst was strikingly manifested by Jesus at the end of his ordeal when he said, "I thirst" (John 19:28). They immediately gave him vinegar to drink, after which he died.

I have been a full time pathologist-medical examiner for many years and I have not come across the terms *postmortem caloricity* or *postmortem fever* used by Kohlbeck and Nitowski. I checked every forensic text in the library of the medical examiner's office, checked with many of my colleagues and initiated a computer search of twenty years of medical and scientific journals to no avail. Although there were many papers dealing with body cooling after death, the only paper in which a study of elevated temperatures were conducted postmortem relating to hyperthermia was one by Hutchins in *Human Pathology* in 1985 in which all the temperatures were taken rectally. He found an initial postmortem increase in temperature measured rectally probably due to an increase in bacterial metabolism without any heat dispersal mechanism but did not measure skin temperatures. I have also confirmed this, but in all the cases of elevated rectal temperatures that I have investigated, in no instance was the skin temperature elevated. If the deceased with an elevated rectal postmortem temperature was found in a cool area, the skin was also cool despite the elevated internal temperature. Moreover, of the thousands of cases we have investigated, we regularly do internal temperatures, yet I have never observed or even heard of a single case where the body temperature was elevated five or six degrees above that maintained at death as indicated by the authors. It is a known fact in forensic pathology that the decedent's exterior (skin) reaches environmental temperature much more rapidly than does his interior. Also, the smaller the body mass, the cooler the environmental temperature and the fewer clothes wrapping the body, the more rapid the cooling time.

Dr. I. Ziderman of the Israel Fiber Institute calls Kohlbeck and Nitowski's hypothesis untenable because mercerization requires highly concentrated alkali solution and near-freezing temperatures (it would be stopped by heat). Also, the acetic acid added for acid sweat would neutralize the slight alkalinity (*Biblical Archaeology Review*: 13:63, 1987).

OTHER STUDIES

POLLEN IDENTIFICATION

Recent studies of pollens found on the Shroud and archaeological comments on the weave pattern have also contributed to estimating the age of the Shroud. These studies were made by Dr. Max Frei, an internationally acclaimed criminalist, who died suddenly in January of 1983. In addition to being Professor of Criminology at the University of Zurich and the founder and a past director of the Zurich Police Scientific Laboratory, he held a doctorate in botany and was a recognized botanical expert regarding the Mediterranean flora.

In 1973, Frei removed dust samples from various locations on the Shroud by means of adhesive tapes and analyzed this dust using a light microscope and a scanning electron microscope. He successfully identified forty-nine species of pollen. In 1978, he removed additional samples from the Shroud and was given samples

FIGURE 12-24

Species of Pollen Found on Shroud *(Courtesy of Professor Werner Bulst.)*

* Places where pollens have been found by Dr. Frei • Other areas where the same plants grow Alphabetical list of the plants whose pollens have been found on the Shroud	France / Italy	Mediterranean Area	Constantinople	Urfa (Edessa)	Jerusalem	Iran / Turin	Arabia / Sahara	Areas of North Africa
1 Acacia albida Del.					*			•
2 Alnus glutinosa Vill.	*							
3 Althaea officinalis L.	*	*			*	•		
4 Amaranthus lividus L.	*	*						
5 Anabasis aphylla L.					*	•	•	•
6 Anemone coronaria L.		*			*			
7 Artemisia Herba-alba Asso				*	*	•	•	•
8 Atraphaxis spinosa L.					*	•		
9 Bassia muricata Asch.					*	•		•
10 Capparis spec.		*		*	*	•		
11 Carduus personata Jacq.	*							
12 Carpinus Betulus L.	*							
13 Cedrus libanotica Lk.	*	*	*		*			
14 Cistus creticus L.		*			*			
15 Corylus avellana L.	*		*					
16 Cupressus sempervirens L.	*	*	*		*			
17 Echinops glaberrimus DC.					*			•
18 Epimedium pubigerum DC.			*					
19 Fagonia mollis Del.					*		•	
20 Fagus silvatica L.	*							
21 Glaucium grandiflorum B & H				*	*	•		
22 Gundelia Tournefortii L.				*	*	•		
23 Haloxylon persicum Bg.					*	•		
24 Haplophyllum tuberculatum Juss.				*	*		•	
25 Helianthemum vesicarium B.					*	•		•

* Places where pollens have been found by Dr. Frei • Other areas where the same plants grow Alphabetical list of the plants whose pollens have been found on the Shroud	France / Italy	Mediterranean Area	Constantinople	Urfa (Edessa)	Jerusalem	Iran / Turin	Arabia / Sahara	Areas of North Africa
26 Hyoscamus aureus L.						*	•	
27 Hyoscamus reticulatus L.					*	*	•	
28 Ixolirion montanum Herb.					*	*		
29 Juniperus oxicedrus L.			*			*	•	
30 Laurus nobilis L.	*	*	*		*			
31 Linum mucronatum Bert.					*	*	•	
32 Lythrum salicaria L.	*							
33 Oligomerus subulata Boiss.			*			*	•	•
34 Onosma syriacum Labill.						*	•	
35 Oryza sativa L.	*							
36 Paliurus spina Christi Mill.		*				*	•	
37 Peganum harmala L.					*	*	•	•
38 Phillyrea angustifolia L.		*				*		
39 Pinus halepensis L.		*				*		
40 Pistacia lentiscus L.		*				*		
41 Pistacia vera L.		*				*		
42 Platanus orientalis L.	*	*	*	*	*	•		
43 Poterium spinosum		*	*			*		
44 Prosopis farcta Macbr.				*	*	•		
45 Prunus spartioides Spach.					*	•		
46 Pteranthus dichotomus Forsk.					*	*	•	
47 Reaumuria hirtella J. & Sp.					*	•	•	
48 Ricinus communis L.	*	*	*	*	*			
49 Ridolfia segetum Moris		*				*		
50 Roemeria hybrida DC.				*	*	*		
51 Scabiosa prolifera L.					*	*		

* Places where pollens have been found by Dr. Frei • Other areas where the same plants grow <hr>Alphabetical list of the plants whose pollens have been found on the Shroud	France / Italy	Mediterranean Area	Constantinople	Urfa (Edessa)	Jerusalem	Iran / Turin	Arabia / Sahara	Areas of North Africa
52 Scirpus triquetus L.	*		*		*			
53 Secale montanum Guss.	*							•
54 Silene conoida L.		*		*	*			
55 Suaeda aegyptiaca Zoh.					*		•	
56 Tamarix nilotica Bunge					*		•	
57 Taxus baccata L.	*		*					
58 Zyglophyllum dumosum Boiss.					*		•	
Total numbers	17	18	13	18	45	25	8	9

from the silver receptacle the Shroud had been stored in. He successfully identified an additional eight species bringing the total up to fifty-eight species (Figure 12-24).

In order to understand the significance of these findings, a brief review of the field of palinology (pollen studies) will be given. Pollens vary in size from ten to two hundred thousandths of a millimeter (one inch equals twenty-five millimeters) and they vary in shape from spherical to spiral and are irregular to smooth in appearance. A protective membrane, called the *esina* is present and is very resistant to chemical action accounting for their excellent preservation under adverse conditions. These pollens mingle in the atmosphere, are carried by air masses, and fall to the earth; when they fall in lakes they settle in layers.

Frei found that only seventeen of the fifty-eight species grew in France or Italy. Practically all the rest were of non-European origin and grew in the Jerusalem area. It is of interest that one of the pollens found on the Shroud derives from the Syrian Christ's Thorn, *Paliurus spina Christi, Mill.* (Figure 12-25), one of the plants believed to be the source of the crown of thorns (see Chapter 3). While some individuals argue that strong winds could carry the pollens from the Jerusalem area to Europe, this is easy to refute. First, the Shroud had only been on exposition for a few days and to say that strong winds arising from Jerusalem carried pollens to the

Shroud exactly on the days of exposition would be too farfetched to carry any scientific weight. Second, since the various pollens bloom at different times of the year, it would be improbable that strong winds could have carried these pollens to the Shroud at such precise times. The studies of Frei certainly offer strong evidence that the Shroud did reside for an extensive period in the Jerusalem area.

It is of interest that many of these pollens have been found embedded as microfossils in the mud at the bottom of the Dead Sea and Lake Gennesareth by Israeli scientists.

Frei also found that none of the pollens were glued to the cloth or covered with tempera adding strong evidence against the Shroud being a painted fake. If his findings prove correct, the supposition that the Shroud was in the Holy Land would be supported. Other specialists, including Dr. Avinoam Danin from the Department of Botany of the Hebrew University in Jerusalem, and a specialist in the desert flora of Israel, studied some of Frei's slides and concurred with his findings, according to Mr. Paul Maloney, Project Director of the Association of Scientists and Scholars International for the Shroud of Turin.

TEXTILE ARCHAEOLOGY

The Shroud consists of a three-to-one handspun, reversing twill, herringbone pattern (Figure 12-25) in which the yarn had been spun with a "Z" twist. Studies of a six to seven centimeter piece from the Shroud by Professor Gilbert Raes of the Meulemeester Technical Laboratory of Textiles of the University of Ghent found unexpected traces of cotton of the species *Gossypium herbaceum* among the linen (Figure 12-26). This presented no difficulty because both linen and cotton were in use in the Middle East at the time of Jesus. According to John Tyrer, a chartered textile technologist of international repute, it is most likely that the Shroud linen is a product of the Middle East since it had not been widely cultivated in Europe. Professor Bollone of the Institute of Forensic Medicine in Turin asserted that weavers at the time of Jesus were in the habit of changing yarns on the same loom. Indeed, it had been argued that the regularity of yarn on the Shroud was indicative of a post-first-century date. But John Tyrer argued that this was not so since the yarns of many ancient Egyptian textiles in Manchester and Halifax museums are even

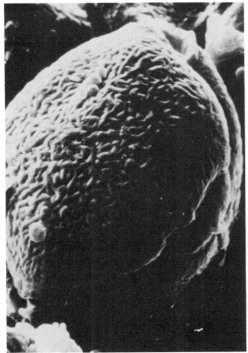

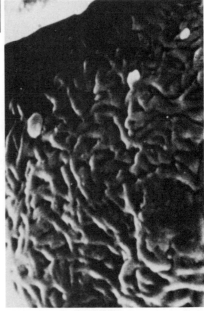

Figure 12-25

Pollen of Paliurus spina Christi Mill.
Found on Shroud by Dr. Max Frei. Magnification: (a) 6,800 times and (b) 12,400 times. (Courtesy of Professor Werner Bulst.)

more regular than the Shroud and that the knowledge and skill of the spanner is the most important consideration. It has also been argued that the Egyptians spun their yarns to afford an "S" twist, not a "Z" twist, but Tyrer points out that "Z" twist yarns have been dated to the late Bronze age and that three-to-one reversing twill could have been produced in first-century Syria or Palestine as they had been at the crossroads of world trade routes.

Many people are amazed to learn that the Turin Shroud is almost two thousand years old and still well preserved. This convinced many that the Shroud could not have survived from the first century. Yet a visit to an Egyptian museum would quickly remove all doubts. Many linen pieces, including mummy cloths, are much older than the Shroud. One is even purported to be almost five thousand years old. Tyre indicates that much older linen fabrics, including Tutankhamun's curtains, are extant and that a publication by Pietro Savio contains an illustration of a cloth woven in a herringbone pattern, dated A.D. 130 that had been excavated by Gayet in the necropolis of Antinoe. Both Professor Raes and Professor Silvio Curto, curator of the Egyptian Museum of Turin, agree that the Shroud probably dates to the time of Jesus. Moreover, Professor Etrano Morano, Director of the Center of Electron Microscopy, studied fibers from the Shroud and compared them with fibers from Egyptian linen more than 2,000 years old using a scanning electron microscope (an instrument that magnifies objects to extremely high magnifications). His investigation reveals "an extraordinary similarity of the surfaces of the Egyptian linen . . . exactly datable beyond 2000 years." He also found pollens between the fibers on both linens, some of which appeared similar.

One area currently under careful scrutiny concerns the identification and reason for the edging strip, the narrow strip of material that divides the main area by a seamlike thickening along the edge of one of the long sides of the Shroud which is joined by sewing thread and displays the same coloration as the main area. A long list of interpretations for the edging strip have been given including the following: it may have been used as a piece that was added to the Shroud to center the image better, or it may have been used as a strengthening band to hang the cloth for displaying the image, or for various uses, to assist in the weaving of the Shroud. The primary reason in identifying this extra edging derives from whether one could use Raes sample for carbon-14 dating. This could have

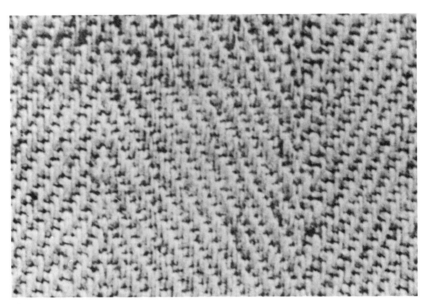

Figure 12-26
Weave of Shroud of Turin.
Magnified several times. Note three in one herringbone weave.

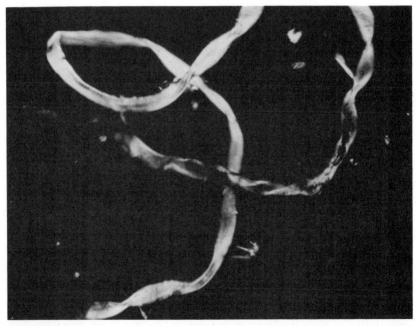

Figure 12-27
Cotton fiber from Shroud of Turin.
Cotton fiber found on sticky tape from blood image area.

serious consequences since it might be a medieval patch of some sort that may have been added on later.

CARBON-14 DATING

Throughout the years, there has been constant reference to carbon-14 dating of the Shroud of Turin as the ultimate scientific proof of its age and the one test that will settle the question of *authenticity* once and for all. Unfortunately, it's not that simple. The method has limitations because cosmic ray and solar variations plus the question of contamination can cause problems in accurately dating the cloth. Yet the experts feel that a reasonably accurate dating is possible.

Carbon-14 (radiocarbon) dating was first described by Nobel Prize winner Willard F. Libby in 1947, who developed it for archaeological and geological dating. The theory behind carbon-14 dating is as follows: Carbon-14 is formed in the earth's atmosphere by the interaction of neutrons with nitrogen-14. These neutrons are produced by an interaction of cosmic rays with the nitrogen in the earth's atmosphere. The carbon-14 is then oxidized to the dioxide and along with carbon-12 and carbon-13 is distributed in the atmosphere, oceans, lakes, etc. Carbon-14 is heavier than normal carbon and begins to decay immediately after it is formed. Under ideal theoretical conditions this decay—in the form of radioactivity—will occur at an exponentially uniform and exact rate. The rate of decay is given in terms of its half-life, the time that is half gone (5,730 years). After this period of time, it continues to lose half of the remainder each 5,730 years, and can be used to date a once living material for up to about 50,000 years and not less than 500 years. The older the sample, the more difficult it is to date because less carbon-14 is present. Under such conditions a larger sample is required for greater accuracy. Conversely, the younger the artifact, the more carbon-14 present, and the smaller the sample required.

The original method is based on the fact that plants take up the carbon 14-dioxide along with nonradioactive carbon dioxide through photosynthesis, and when animals eat plants, the carbon-14 is incorporated in their tissues. When the organism dies, it immediately stops taking in the carbon-14 and begins to lose this radioactive carbon at the rate indicated above. The original technique of dating required burning the object to form carbon dioxide, which was then purified and chemically reduced to pure carbon by hot magnesium. The amount of radioactivity is then measured with a Geiger counter that counts the radioactive rays given off. Libby's original method required a relatively large sample: in the case of the Shroud a piece as big as a large handkerchief. Newer methods have evolved for performing the test on small samples, even as small as a single eight inch piece of thread. Two carbon-14 techniques are currently being used: the *proportional gas counter method* and the *accelerator mass spectrometry method*. The small proportional counter method, which may require several weeks, is a modified conventional technique that measures the decay products of carbon-14. The accelerator mass spectrometry method is a newly developed method that actually counts the carbon-14 atoms rather than the beta rays after causing a high energy acceleration of the ions and sequentially removing all but the carbon-14 ions. It is a revolutionary method because it utilizes very tiny samples, can purportedly extend the measurement time beyond 50,000 years, can perform the test in hours, and is allegedly (though there is some disagreement) more accurate than conventional methods.

Carbon-14 dating was denied in 1976 by the special commission appointed by Cardinal Pelligrino, archbishop of Turin, because it was felt that a sizable portion of the Shroud would have to be destroyed. Later, when it was established that accurate dating could be performed on very small samples, the commission agreed to have six radiocarbon laboratories perform a small sample dating test on known ancient fabrics. The British Museum was chosen to act as independent coordinator. In May of 1983, two samples, one Egyptian linen from about B.C. 3000 and one Peruvian cotton from about A.D. 1200, and later an additional sample, Peruvian cotton from about A.D. 1000–1400, each piece weighing 100 milligrams, were submitted to the radiocarbon accelerator laboratories at the University of Tucson (Arizona), University of Rochester (New York), Oxford University (England), and Zurich (Switzerland), and to the small gas counter laboratories at Brookhaven (New York) and Harwell (England). The laboratories knew the source but did not know the ages of the samples. The results were presented at the 12th International Radio Carbon Dating Conference at Trodhein, Norway, on June 12, 1985, and indicated good agreement between the laboratories and offered no differences between the accelerator and small counter laboratories. These studies have now set the stage for an attempt to date the Shroud of Turin.

The question of accuracy of the method relates primarily to variations in carbon-14 production and the inherent contamination problems. In the first instance, the variations in carbon-14 production appear to be related to factors influencing incoming cosmic radiations such as the magnetic field of the earth and solar changes. Dr. Minze Stuiver and his group from the University of Washington have made great strides in correcting for these atmospheric factors. They developed carbon-14 calibration curves using tree fragments in which the calendar ages have been determined by the science of dendrochronology. In this science dating is determined by studying growth patterns in tree rings, using species that live for long periods such as California Sequoias and Bristlecone pines.

The second problem, contamination, is important because samples contaminated with modern carbon can make a sample appear hundreds or even thousands of years younger. William Meacham, an anthropologist from the University of Hong Kong, expressed concern about the accuracy of carbon-14 dating in the June 1986 edition of *Shroud Spectrum International*. In his article, he warned that there was a period of about 600 years during which the Shroud was subjected to many different environments and uncertain handling situations and during which a long list of contaminants may have been introduced by man. He also pointed out the possibility of an additional 1,300 years in which the Shroud might have been in contact with a host of other contaminating conditions. He specifically argued that neither the Raes sample nor the charred portions can be relied on for carbon-14 dating and that specific care in identifying and decontaminating all contaminants must be attempted. He further suggested that carbon-14 experts who regularly do carbon-14 testing must be consulted for a full investigation of this test. The experts, however, who will participate in this test are the best in the world, are completely aware of the problems inherent to the test, are meticulously taking all precautions regarding variations and contamination, and appear confident that they will arrive at an accurate calendrical date.

COINS OVER THE EYES

The first report of images consistent with coinlike objects found over the eyes of the Turin image came from the three-dimensional computer studies of Jumper and Jackson in 1977.

Using a VP-8 image analyzer, these investigators noted buttonlike objects over both eyes in a three-dimensional shape of coins. They researched the literature and found references to early Jewish customs that showed that coins or potsherd were placed over the eyes of deceased individuals to prevent them from viewing the way to their final place in eternity.

After hearing this, Reverend Francis Filas, a Jesuit theologian from Loyola University, feverishly delved into an intensive study of the eye area (Figure 12-28a) and in collaboration with Michael Marx, a numismatist from Chicago, reported in 1980 that certain photographic markings over the eyes revealed a striking similarity to those found on lepton coins (widow mites) issued during the reign of Pontius Pilate between the years A.D. 29 and 32 (Figure 12-29b). These markings appear to depict an astrologer's staff (*lituus*) and four Greek letters, UCAI, angling around the crook of the staff at 9:30 to 11:30 o'clock (Figure 12-29a). This is believed to represent part of the coin inscription, TIBERIOUKAICAROC, which translates "of Tiberius Caesar." Measuring and comparing the photographic image over the right eye with those of an actual Pilate coin, Marx found a consistency ". . . of size, position, angular rotation, relative mutual proportion, accuracy of duplication (with an exception of "C" on the Shroud where a "K" is present on Pilate coins we possess)." Filas indicated that, with mathematical probability, there would be one chance in 6.22×10^{42} that the markings on the eyes are a random occurrence.

In 1981, Filas enlisted the help of Log E/Interpretations Systems to subject the Shroud image to sophisticated computer image analysis. A three-dimensional image was produced that strikingly demonstrated both the staff and the letters UCAI (Figure 28b). Several numismatic experts disputed Filas' findings primarily on the basis of the "C" for "K" error, and on the dating in general but the debate simmered down markedly when Filas located a few Pilate coins that showed a minting error of a "C" for a "K." Later Alan and Mary Whanger from Duke University Medical Center developed a polarized image overlay technique in which two images, one of a computer enhanced photograph of the right eye region and the other of the coin used by Filas, were projected through polarizing filters onto a screen and a fine details comparison was made. They reported an almost perfect match with seventy-four points of congruence with all the letters UCAI and indicated that they identified the remainder of the eroded letters, TIOU/CAICAROC, with a reasonable degree of certainty. They also reported that the image on the left eye was less distinct but claim that the image coincided with another Pontius Pilate lepton known in numismatic circles as the "Julia lepton" struck only in A.D. 29, with seventy-three points of congruence.

Further support for Filas' hypothesis was provided by Dr. Robert Haralick, director of the Spatial Data Analysis Laboratory at Virginia Polytechnic Institute and State University at Blackburg, Virginia. Using digital image analysis of the negative image over the right eye, he reported the finding of two additional letters, an "O" and a "C", before and after the UCAI.

What is the mechanism for such image formation? One suggestion was made by Dr. Igor Benson, an engineer and Russian Orthodox priest from North Carolina who has been studying the effect of radiation from high voltage, high frequency electrical discharges. Benson suggests that ball lightning might have been the culprit, striking the body during an electrical storm, charging it with high voltage energy, which would have immediately dissipated its ionic energy (discharge), thus scorching the cloth. He provided an experimental model by directing a high energy source from a cathode energy tube located within a glass ball to a small coin placed on a piece of linen in the energy field. A scorch occurred on the linen showing fine details of the coin. Dr. Scheuermann, a physicist from Germany, and Dr. Graeme Coote, a physicist from New Zealand, have also been involved independently in the question of high voltage electrical discharges producing the image on the Shroud. Coote, however, is of the opinion that the high voltages may have been produced from stresses on rock during an earthquake rather than from ball lightning as proposed by Benson (see section, *"Electrical Discharge Modification"* under *"The Scorch Theory"*).

The importance of the coin hypothesis is certainly self-evident relative to dating the Shroud. If this hypothesis was determined valid, it would date the Shroud image right to the time of Jesus. Unfortunately, many scientists are not convinced, arguing that these supposed coin images are natural occurrences resulting from the coarseness of the fiber weave. Perhaps more precise photographic techniques of the eye region made both at close range and with increased magnification using appropriate filters may resolve

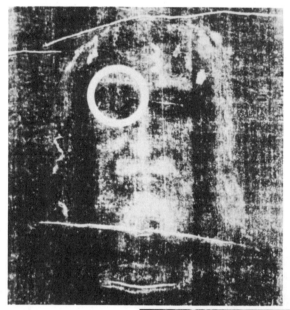

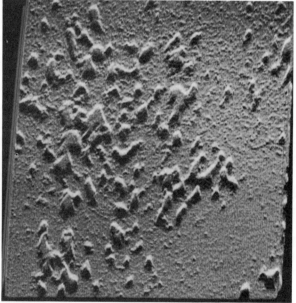

Figure 12-28

Head region of the Shroud of Turin (a) and 3-D relief of right eye region (b).

(a) White circle indicates right eye region where Roman coin was allegedly placed over the eye.

(b) Letters "UCAI" in upper left from 10 to 11 o'clock is believed to represent some of the letters on the Pilate lepton depicted in Figure 12-29b. The astrologer's staff (lituus) is also seen to the left of center. (See text.)

By Francis Filas, S.J. (Courtesy of Peter D. Fox, S.J., Loyola University.)

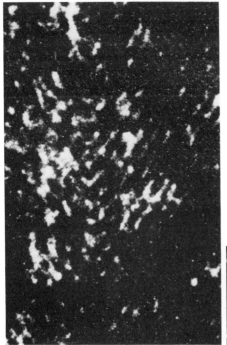

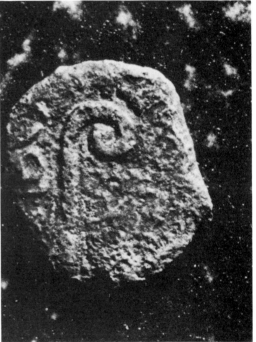

Figure 12-29

Shroud of Turin, blowup of right eye area (a) and a typical Pontius Pilate lepton existing today (b).

(a) The letters "UCAI" and the astrologer's staff are again noted in the right eye region.

(b) the astrologer's staff is upright and the letters are located in the left upper region of the lepton. The size is one half inch (12 millimeters). It is at the same magnification as the image in (a). Compare the two and refer to the text.

By Francis Filas, S.J. (Courtesy of Peter D. Fox, S.J., Loyola University.)

this controversy. Moreover, samples of fibrils from the eye region may show traces of copper when examined by histochemical, or spectroscopic analysis.

BLOOD STUDIES

The puce-colored areas on the wound areas of the Turin Shroud purported to be blood stand out in marked contrast to the sepia tones of the image of the man of the Shroud. There is little question that these areas strikingly resemble the appearance of blood and in general correspond directly to the various wounds suffered during the scourging, crowning with thorns, and crucifixion. Scientific studies of the "blood stained areas" were first conducted in 1973, after a special group of experts, the Turin Commission, was first convened in 1969 to examine and conduct tests on the Shroud and make special recommendations for further scientific testing. In 1973 Professor Giorgio Franche, a serologist and director of the Institute of Legal Medicine, University of Modena, ran chemical tests for blood on ten separate threads from "blood"-stained areas of the Shroud that proved negative. In the same year, Professors Guido Filogamo and Alberto Zina, ordinaries in human anatomy, University of Turin, were unable to find evidence of blood on the threads under the electron microscope. They indicated that rarely can blood traces be positively isolated unless they are of recent origin, and both scientists, however, have admitted that their negative findings do not exclude the possibility of blood. Up until 1980, however, there had been no confirmation, chemically or morphologically, that these areas were blood.

In 1980, Drs. Alan Adler and John Heller, using time consuming spectroscopic and microchemical tests, reported the presence of blood on linen fibrils from sticky tape samples taken from the wound areas of the Shroud (Figure 12-30). Dr. Baima Bollone independently confirmed this finding and with Jorio and Massaro also demonstrated, using a fluorescent antibody technique, that the blood was of human origin. The latter group later reported the successful typing of the blood as type AB, but this finding is controversial. Many forensic serologists are unconvinced of the ability to type archaeological specimens of this type, particularly since the Shroud was in such a hot fire at Chambéry. *Therefore, the question of blood-typing must be held in abeyance since no adequate*

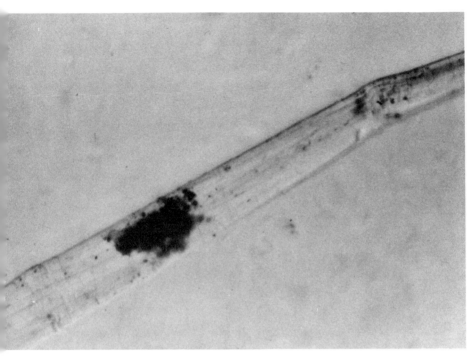

Figure 12-30
Linen fibril from Shroud of Turin.
Sticky tape from blood image area. The dark area is believed to be blood.

studies have yet been published in the scientific literature confirming the accuracy of typing archaeological blood specimens.

Forensic studies were also conducted in 1970 on the blood and tissue relics of Lanciano* by a group of medical specialists. These relics were alleged to be type AB.

It is also important to realize that the presence of blood in the blood image areas of the Shroud does not completely preclude artifice. A clever artist who is trying to deceive the public might have actually used blood on the wound areas.

---

*According to legend, in the eighth century, while saying mass, a priest doubted that he was converting the bread and wine into the body and blood of Jesus. Before his very eyes, the bread changed into flesh and the wine into blood. Both species were kept in separate reliquaries and venerated since that time. In 1970, a group of medical experts tested these samples using sophisticated forensic techniques. *They concluded that the 'blood' was type AB human blood and the 'flesh' was human heart muscle.*

CONCLUSIONS AND FUTURE CONSIDERATIONS

The authenticity of the Shroud of Turin has been one of the greatest riddles in history. Centuries have passed and the battle still rages. One fact is certain: if the various specimens of antiquity now in museums all over the world were subjected to the same scientific scrutiny as the Shroud only a few pieces would survive.

Although much new information has been gleaned from the scientific studies on the Shroud after the 1978 exposition, the mechanism by which the image was created is still a mystery. Some of the new information is as follows: The yellow coloration of the body only image appears to be due to an accelerated aging process as compared to the nonimage areas and caused by a dehydration, oxidation, and conjugation effect. This body image is only present in the surface fibrils and appears to be absent around the periphery of blood image areas. This suggests that the blood images and the body only image were the result of two independent processes: the blood being laid down first by direct contact, and then the image by some type of projection process causing linen degradation in a cloth-body distance relationship. The blood image areas were determined to contain blood consistent with human blood.

The report of iron oxide, vermillion, tempera, and traces of other artist pigments by Walter McCrone, an internationally renowned microscopist, rekindled the artistic theory that began with the famous D'Arcy memorandum, which stated the Shroud had been painted by a cunning artist and that the artist had been found. Chemical, optical, computer and other recently published investigations, however, refute McCrone's findings and indicate that there was not enough iron oxide to account for the image, that the image did not afford a spectroscopic picture consistent with iron oxide, that the x-ray studies were not consistent with iron oxide, and that, although there were tiny amounts of iron oxide on the Shroud, most of the iron was due to an ion association effect of the linen in trapping iron during the retting process. Moreover, there was no evidence of paints, dyes, or pigments on the Shroud, and recent studies do indicate that many shrouds have been painted by artists, sometimes in the same room. Sometimes the shrouds were laid flat on top of the Turin Shroud to make relics, thus very probably accounting for traces of artist's paints on the Shroud of

Turin. Computer studies resulted in a vivid, three-dimensional production of the Shroud showing that a cloth-body distance effect must have been active. Filas' report identified the coin over the right eye as a Roman coin, a Pilate lepton dating to A.D. 28–30, and supported by Whanger's polarization-overlay technique. The pollen studies of Frei have added additional weight to the Shroud being a first century relic, even though many scientists still question the validity of his methodology. Thus, overall, there is still much controversy about authenticity, but a great deal of new information has emerged. The overwhelming consensus of opinion on both sides demands careful carbon-14 studies to date the Shroud.

Controversies relating to authenticity and the inability to determine the cause of the Shroud image have led to intensive demands on the Turin authorities and the Holy See in Rome to allow for carbon-14 dating and perhaps other forms of testing. Although initially denied because of a fear of damage to the Shroud, and later by fear of inaccuracy of the techniques in radiocarbon dating, testing has finally been approved for the winter of 1987 by Cardinal Ballestrero of Turin, Umberto di Savoia (who agreed prior to his death in 1983), and Pope John Paul II. This approval came after a trial run to date samples of ancient textiles by several radiocarbon accelerator and proportional gas counter laboratories demonstrated comparative and accurate results. Professor Carlos Chagas, president of the Pontifical Academy of Sciences, organized a four-day conference to establish a protocol for carrying out the carbon-14 dating. Areas discussed included: where to remove samples from the Shroud to avoid problems with contamination, who would remove the samples, who would oversee the tests, and what radiocarbon laboratories would perform the tests. The laboratories selected included five accelerator laboratories at Oxford directed by Professor Hall, the University of Arizona directed by Professor Donahue, CRNS, France directed by Professor Duplessy, and the University of Rochester directed by Professor Gove. Two proportional gas counter laboratories in Harwell, England, directed by Professor Otlet and Brookhaven Laboratories in New York, directed by Professor Harbottle, were also chosen. The British Museum will oversee the entire operation by maintaining the samples, submitting blind samples consisting of Shroud and non-Shroud samples to all of the laboratories, and submitting the

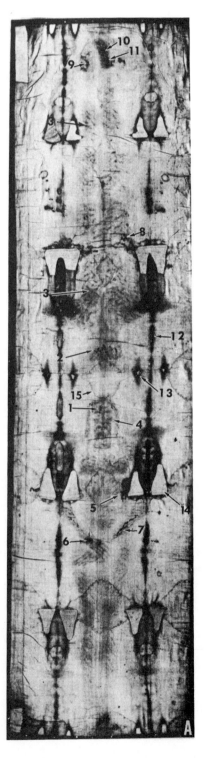

Figure 12-31

Diagram of the entire Shroud of Turin.
The entire front and back are shown.
(a) *The Shroud as observed by the naked eye (right is left and vice versa).*
(b) *The negative image of the Shroud. Note that the negative image is striking and shows a complete inversion of light values. The Shroud as we view it appears to be an almost perfect negative.*
1) *Blood stains on forehead from thorns*
2) *Blood stains on back of head from crown*
3) *Scourge marks*
4) *Swelling on right cheek*
5) *Wound of side (spear)*
6) *Nail wound of hand*
7) *Blood stains on the forearm*
8) *Continuation of blood from chest wound (5)*
9) *Left heel*
10) *Nail wound of foot*
11) *Right sole and heel*
12) *Burns along folds*
13) *Holes from molten silver*
14) *Patches sewn by Poor Clares*
15) *Water stains*
(Nos. 12–15 caused by Chambéry fire in 1532)

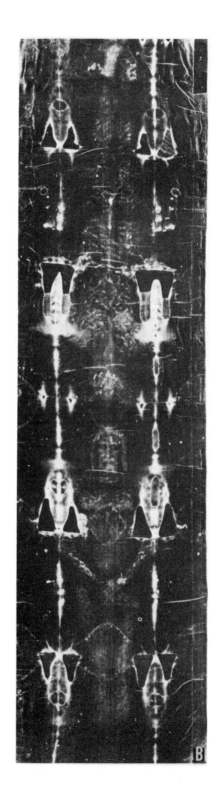

results to the proper authorities in Turin. It has also granted approval for a team of scientists and scholars to perform some additional tests on the Shroud, although when and what examinations will be allowed are currently secret. A deadline of Easter, 1988 has been tentatively agreed on for final results of all tests.

Many critics have questioned why additional tests need be conducted if radiocarbon dating places the Shroud in the middle ages? The reason is clear. Even if the radiocarbon tests date the Shroud no earlier than the thirteenth century, the *cause* of the image has still evaded us throughout the centuries, and even space-age sophisticated analyses have not solved the mystery. If it were done by artifice, it would constitute one of the greatest, if not the greatest, perpetrations of fraud in history. Therefore the solution to the "riddle of the Shroud" would finally be put to rest. If, on the other hand, the Shroud is dated to the first century, there would be three possibilities: it is the Shroud of Jesus; it is a shroud of a man crucified at the time of Jesus or within a possible 150 year spread (if there are no complications in radiocarbon dating), or it is an artistic copy done in the first century or in medieval times on a piece of linen from the first century. If the artistic theory can be put to rest by additional information gleaned from subsequent tests, we still would not have a test for Jesus, as Adler so aptly pointed out, but the information would favor it being the Shroud of Jesus because of the presence of the image depicting the crown of thorns, the spear wound image, the absence of the *crurifracium*, but most importantly because of the absence of decomposition. A shroud normally would never be removed from the corpse of a crucified person, thus remaining on the corpse throughout decomposition and either decomposing with the body or being severely stained and rotted. This was not so with Jesus because he only remained in the Shroud for about thirty-four to thirty-six hours after being placed on it. Moreover, if subsequent testing confirmed the validity of the coin hypothesis of Filas and the pollen studies of Frei, the evidence would be overwhelmingly in favor of authenticity. If this proves true, there would no longer be a Shroud of Turin but instead. . . . . the *Shroud of Jesus*.

13

Recapitulation

In the preceding chapters, I have attempted to analyze critically the sufferings of Christ and the mechanism of death from Gethsemane to Calvary. Now let us summarize the journey from his Agony in the Garden to his ignominious death on the cross.

"My soul is sorrowful, even unto death, remain here and watch" (Mark 14:34). Jesus was totally aware of all the sufferings that would come during the next day. Suddenly, his heart began to pound thunderously against his chest at a rapid rate, his color became ashen, his pupils dilated, and his breathing became very rapid. Adrenalin was being pumped throughout his body; the fight or flight reaction had been enacted. The severe mental anguish of his sufferings to come had begun, draining the strength from his body. He fell to the ground and prayed over and over again, then looked up to heaven, " 'Father, if thou art willing, remove this cup from me, nevertheless not my will but yours be done.' And there appeared to him an angel from heaven strengthening him, and being in agony he prayed more earnestly and his sweat became like drops of blood falling upon the ground" (Luke 22:42–44). He had accepted his fate. Now his heart rate began to slow, his face became flushed, his muscles relaxed, and his body became drenched with sweat as clots of blood dropped to the ground from small hemorrhages into his sweat glands. Jesus became limp from extreme exhaustion.

Later, he was taken before the Sanhedrin, where he was accused of blasphemy and then brought before Pilate and accused of "perverting our nation and forbidding us to give tribute to Caesar, saying that he himself is Christ the King" (Luke 23:1–2). But neither Pilate nor Herod could find fault in this man.

"Then Pilate therefore took Jesus, and scourged *him*" (John 19:1). Jesus was bent over and tied to a low pillar, where he was flogged across the back, chest, and legs with a multifaceted flagrum with bits of metal on the ends. Over and over again the metal tips dug deep into the flesh, ripping small vessels, nerves, muscles, and skin. His body became distorted with pain, causing him to fall to the ground, only to be jerked up again. Seizurelike activities occurred, followed by tremors, vomiting, and cold sweats. Screams echoed out at the conclusion of each stroke. His mouth was dry, and his tongue stuck to the roof of his mouth.

Unfortunately, the scourging was initiated by the Romans so that the Deuteronomic limit of forty lashes less one was not followed. He was reduced to a wretched state because Pilate wanted to appease the mob so they would not demand that he crucify Jesus. This did not appease them. They were after blood, as they cried out, " 'Crucify him.' The soldiers clothed him with a purple cloak and plaiting a crown of thorns put it on him and began to salute him" (Mark 15:17–19). They took the Syrian Christ thorn, which was growing at the side of the praetorium, fashioned it into a cap by interweaving it, and placed it on his head. This was the royal crown for the King of the Jews, and a reed was his royal scepter. They paid homage to the new king as they filed past, kneeling and then striking him across the face with the scepter and spitting on him. His cheeks and nose became reddened, bruised, and swollen, and stabbing pains that felt like electric shocks or red hot pokers traversed his face, immobilizing him so he was afraid to turn lest the pain might reoccur. His face became distorted, and Jesus tensed his whole body so that he would not move, for every movement activated little trigger zones, bringing on agonizing attacks.

Pilate then ordered Jesus crucified, and the centurion and his *quaternio* placed the crosspiece weighing over fifty pounds on his shoulders, which had been severely lacerated by the flogging. This brought on bitter pain, throwing him to his knees. The soldiers jerked him back to his feet. People lined both sides of the street with the cohort of soldiers maintaining order as Jesus, in a state of traumatic shock, continued along the uphill route, falling fre-

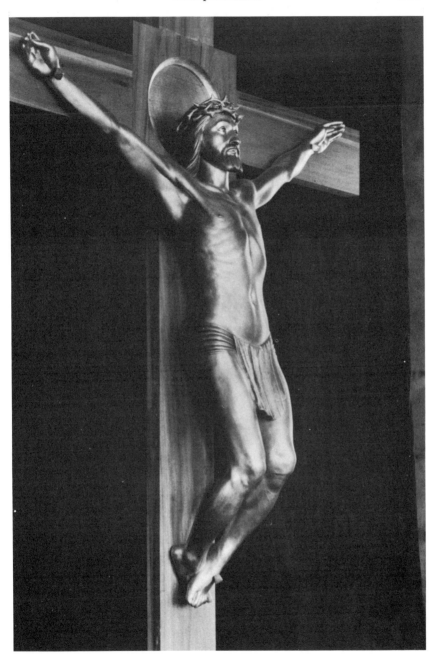

Figure 13-1
Sculptured and bronzed crucifix.
This crucifix was made by the late Father Peter Weyland, SVD, a brilliant and gifted sculptor. The extreme accuracy of position and angle was assured because Father Weyland's assistants poured plaster over his body while he was suspended.

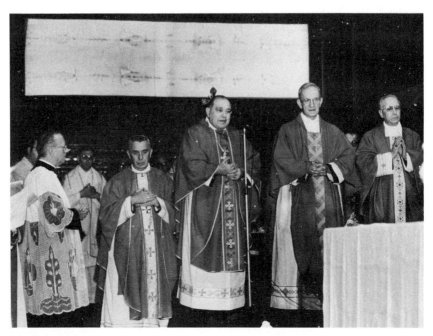

Figure 13-2
Shroud of Turin during public viewing in 1978.
Special masses were said every morning during the Exposition.
(Courtesy of the Reverend Peter M. Rinaldi, S.D.B.)

quently with the crosspiece landing on top of him. The noonday
sun was hot, and the sweat poured from his body, causing severe
thirst. He could not move his tongue, which felt several times its
size. His entire body was reacting to the pain from the multiple
wounds afforded by the scourging. It was easy for the centurion to
see that he would not make it to Calvary at this rate. Therefore, a
visitor to the city, Simon of Cyrene, was called into service to carry
the *patibulum* the rest of the way. Jesus continued to stumble and
fall all the way to Golgotha along the uphill, bumpy, dusty road. At
Calvary the soldiers threw their dice for his vestments, and the
winner found them clotted to the multiple lacerations that were
caused by the flogging. The soldier grasped it at the bottom and
yanked it off. The entire body of Jesus felt as though it was on fire.
The crosspiece was set on the ground, and Jesus was placed on top
of it while three men of the team held him down. A large, square
iron nail was then driven through the palm of the hand just in the

fold of the large muscular prominence at the base of his thumb. How Jesus wrenched and struggled! The pain was unbearable, burning, and incessant. The second hand was then nailed in the same manner. There was no struggle this time, as he became limp. He was then forced to his feet because his knees buckled. Two of the team lifted each end of the *patibulum* while the other two grasped him, helping him to ascend the stairs that were placed in front of the *stipes*. When he reached the top of the steps, the *patibulum* was lifted onto the mortise that had been cut out of the upright. The steps were then pulled away, leaving him suspended by his hands. The two men bent his knees and lifted his heels against the upright until his feet were flush to the cross. As each soldier held a foot, another soldier of the team drove a nail through each one. The pain was bitter, but Christ hardly moved. He did not have the strength to fight. He was almost totally exhausted and in severe pain. Sweat poured over his entire body, drenching him, and his face assumed a yellowish-ashen color. His respirations increased in number, and he twisted and turned, assuming different positions in an attempt to relieve some of his pains. The burning pains from the nails, the lancinating lightning bolts across the face from irritation by the crown of thorns, the excruciating wounds from the scourging, the severe pull on the shoulders, the intense cramps in the knees, and the severe thirst together composed a symphony of unrelenting pain. Then he lifted his head up to heaven and cried out in a loud voice, "It is consummated." Jesus was dead.

References

Accetta, Joseph S. "X-ray Fluorescence Analysis and Infrared Thermography with Applications to the Shroud of Turin." *Proceedings of the 1977 United States Conference of Research on the Shroud of Turin.* Colorado Springs, 1977, pp. 110–23.

Accetta, J. S. and J. S. Baumgart. "Infrared Reflectance Spectroscopy and Thermographic Investigations of the Shroud of Turin." *Applied Optics* 19(12):1921–29.

Adams, F. O. and A. Sindon. *Layman's Guide to the Shroud of Turin.* Tempe, AZ: Synergy Books, 1982.

Adams, L. D. and J. Hope. "Nervousness, Anxiety and Depression." In *Principles of Internal Medicine,* edited by Harrison, J. R., R. Adams, I. L. Bennett, Jr., W. Resnik, G. Thorn, and M. M. Wintrobe. New York: Blakiston Division, McGraw-Hill, 1966.

Adler, Alan. Personal Correspondence, November 5, 1984.

Anderson, W. A. D. and J. M. Kissane. *Pathology.* Saint Louis: C. V. Mosby, 1977.

Angelino, P. F. and M. Abrata. "Dibattito Sulla Morta Fisica Di Gesu." *Sindon,* (December, 1982):11–18.

Asche, Geoffrey. "What Sort of Picture." *Sindon* (1966):15–19.

Avis, C., D. Lynn, J. Lorre, S. Lavoie, J. Clark, E. Armstrong and J. Addington. "Image Processing of the Shroud of Turin. 1982. *Proceedings of the International Conference on Cybernetics and Society.* October, 1982.

P. L. Baima Bollone and A. Gaglio. "Demonstration of Blood. Techniques." *Shroud Spectrum International* No. 13 (1984):3–8.

P. L. Baima Bollone, M. Iorio, and A. L. Massaro. "La dimostrazione della presenze di tracce di sangue umano sulla Sindone." *Sindon* No. 30, (1982).

P. L. Baima Bollone, M. Iorio, and A. L. Massaro. "Identificazione del gruppo delle tracce di sangue umano sulla Sindone." *Sindon* 31 (1982).

P. L. Baima Bollone, M. Iorio, and A. L. Massaro. "Identification of the Group of the Traces of Human Blood in the Shroud." *Shroud Spectrum International,* March No. 6(1983):3–6.

Barasch, M. "The Scientists and the Shroud." *The Catholic Digest,* (April, 1979):100–109.

Barbet, P. *Les cinq plaies du Christ.* Second ed. Paris: Procure du Carmel de l'Action de Graces, 1937.

Barbet, Pierre. *Doctor at Calvary.* New York: P. J. Kennedy & Sons, 1953; New York: Image Books, 1963.

Barnes, Arthur S. *The Holy Shroud of Turin.* London: Burns, Oates and Washbourne, 1934.

Becker, A. E. and J. P. van Mantoem. "Cardiac Tamponade: A Study of 50 Hearts." *European Journal of Cardiology* 3(1975):319–358.

Bedini, D. B. *The Sessorian Relics of the Passion of Our Lord.* Rome: Tipografia Pio X Via Etruschi Imprim, 1956.

Berosma, S. "Did Jesus Die of a Broken Heart? "Calvin Forum 14:(1948)196–167.

Bishop, J. *The Day Christ Died.* New York: Harper & Row, 1957.

Bloomquist, E. R. "A Doctor Looks at Crucifixion." *Christian Herald* 1964:35, 46–48.

Bocca, M., A. Messina, and V. Salvi. "Revisione critica anatomica sulle lesioni della mano e del polso dell'Uomo della Sindone." Second International Congress. The Shroud and Science, Turin, Italy, October 7–8, 1978.

Bollone, P. L. M. "Rilievi e considerazioni medico legali sulla formazione delle immagini sulla Sindone." Second International Congress. "The Shroud and Science, Turin, Italy, October 7–8, 1978.

Bortin, V. "Science and the Shroud of Turin." *Biblical Archaeologist* 43(1980):109–117.

Brandone, A. "L'analisi per attivazione neutronica nello studio della Sindone di Torino." Second International Congress. The Shroud and Science, Turin, Italy, October 7–8, 1978.

Braunwald, E., K. J. Isselbacher, R. G. Petersdorf, J. D. Wilson, J. B. Martin, and A. S. Fauci. *Harrison's Principles of Internal Medicine.* New York: McGraw-Hill, 1987.

Brent, O. and D. Rolfe. *The Silent Witness.* Futura: London, 1978.

Brewer, L. A., B. Burbank, P. C. Sampson and C. A. Schiff. "The Wet Lung in War Casualties." Archives of Surgery, 123(1946):343.

Broeg, L., *Elemental Treatise of Practical Dermatology.* Paris, 1907. (Hematidosis).

Bucklin, Robert. "The Legal and Medical Aspects of the Trial and Death of Christ." *Medicine, Science and the Law* (January 1970):14–26.

Bucklin, Robert. "The Medical Aspects of the Crucifixion of Our Lord Jesus Christ." *Linacre Quarterly* (February 1958).

Bucklin, R. "The Shroud of Turin: Viewpoint of a Forensic Pathologist." *Shroud Spectrum International* 13(1984):3–8.

Bucklin, Robert. "The Pathologist Looks at the Shroud." Second International Congress. The Shroud and Science. Turin, Italy. October 7–8, 1978.

Bulst, Werner. *The Shroud of Turin.* Milwaukee: Bruce, 1957.

———. "The Pollen Grains on the Shroud of Turin." *Shroud Spectrum International* 10(1981):20.

———. "Turiner Grabtuch und Exeoese heute." *Biblische Zeitschrift* (1984):22–42. (Schoninah).

———. "Turiner Grabtuch und Exeoese heute." II. Neues zur Geschichte des Tuches. *Biblische Zeitschrift* (1984):22–42. (Schoninah).

Bulst, W. "The Imprints of the Feet on the Shroud of Turin, a Complex Problem." Personal publication, 1986.

Bulst, W. "Some Considerations on the Genesis of the Body Image on the Shroud of Turin." *Shroud Specturm International* 19(1986):214.

Burden, A. "Shroud of Mystery." *Science* 81(2)(1981):76–83.

Buttrick, G. A. et al. (editors) *The Interpreter's Bible.* Nashville: Abingdon Coberbury Press, 1951.

Camps, F. E. *Gradwohl's Legal Medicine.* Second ed. Baltimore: Williams & Wilkins Co., 1968. (Chapter 19, pp. 345–51).

The Catholic Encyclopedia. New York: Encyclopedia Press, 1913.

Cazzola P. "Il Volto Santo e il Sudario di Cristo (plascanica) nell' arte sacra russa." Second International Congress, The Shroud and Science, Turin, Italy. October 7–8, 1978.

Centro Internazionale di Sindonologia, Osservazioni Alle Perizie Ufficiali sulla santa Sindone, 1969–1976. Via S. Domenico, 28 10122 Torino.

Charrier, Giovanni. "Pollens under the Microscope." *La Sindone,* supplemento de La Stampa Torino 27 Agosto–8 Ottobre 1978.

Cheshire, L. *Pilgrimage to the Shroud.* McGraw-Hill: New York, 1956.

Chippendale, C. "Radiocarbon Comes of Age." *New Scientist,* July 21, 1983.

Clark, C. C. P. "What Was the Physical Cause of the Death of Jesus Christ?" *Medical Record* 38(1890):543.

Condulmer, Piera. *La Sindone* (Testimone o Inganno). Codella Editore Torino, 1978.

Cook, C. "Coin of the Shroud of Turin." *Coinage Magazine* 17(1981):70–74.

Cooper, H. C. "The Agony of Death by Crucifixion." *New York Medical Journal* 38(1883):150–153.

Crawley, Geoffrey. "The Turin Shroud." *British Journal of Photography* (March 24, 1967):228–232.

Crowfoot, G. *Methods of Hand Spinning in Egypt and the Sudan.* Bankfield Museum: Halifax, 1974.

Culliton, Barbara J. "The Mystery of the Shroud of Turin Challenges 20th-Century Science." *Science,* 201(July 21, 1978):235–39.

Dalman, G. *Arbeit und Sitte in Palestina.* Vol. 2, 1928.

Daniels, R. A., Jr., and W. R. Cate., Jr. "Wet Lung—An Experimental Study." *Annals of Surgery* 172(1948):836.

Darier, G. "Hermatidrosis." *Basis of Dermatology.* Moscow-Leningrad Edition, 1930.

Davis, C. T. "The Crucifixion of Jesus. The Passion of Christ from a Medical Point of View." *Arizona Medicine,* March, 1965.

Delage, Yves. "Le Linceul de Turin." *Rome Scientifique* 17(1902):683–87.

Delage, Y. "Le Linceuul de Turin." *Revue Scientifique* 4(ser. 17, 1902):683–687.

DeSalvo, J. A. "The Image Formation Process of the Shroud of Turin and Its Similarities to Volkringer Patterns." *Shroud Spectrum International* 6(1984):7–15.

DePasquale, N. P. and G. E. Burch. "Death by Crucifixion." *American Heart Journal,* 66(1963):434.

Devan, D., and V. Miller. "Quantitative Photographs of the Shroud of Turin." Institute of Electric and Electronics Engineers 1982 *Proceedings of the International Conference on Cybernetics and Society.* October, 1982.

diMaria, A. L. "Saluti e commiato." Second International Congress, The Shroud and Science, Turin, Italy, October 7–8, 1978.

Dinegar, R. H. "The 1978 Scientific Study of the Shroud of Turin." *Shroud Spectrum International* 1(1982):3–12.

Dunphy, J. E. and L. W. Wag. *Surgical Diagnosis and Treatment*. Los Altos, California. Lange Medical Publishing, 1975.

Ecker, Arthur. "Tic Douloureux." *New York State Journal of Medicine*. August (1974):1586–1594.

Edwards, W. D., W. J. Gabel, and F. E. Hosmer. "On the Physical Death of Jesus Christ." *Journal of the American Medical Association*. 255(1986):1455–1463.

Egger, G. "Prova dell'autenticita della Sindone dal punto di vista della *storia* dell' arte." Second International Congress, The Shroud and Science, Turin, Italy. October 7–8, 1978.

Egidi, C., P. Grattoni, and G. Quaglia. "Considerazioni sulla fotografia telemetrica di una statua in relazione con le impronte della sindone." Second International Congress, The Shroud and Science, Turin, Italy, October 7–8, 1978.

Ellis, R. A., W. Montagna, and H. Fanger. "Histology and Cytochemistry of Human Skin XIF: The Blood Supply of the Cutaneous Glands." *Journal of Investigative Dermatology*. 30(1958):137–45.

Enrie, G. *La Sante Sindone rivelata dalla fotografia*. Turin, 1938.

Ercoline, W., R. Downs, Jr., and J. Jackson. "Examination of the Shroud for Image Distortions." Institute of Electric and Electronics Engineers 1982 *Proceedings of the International Conference on Cybernetics and Society*. October, 1982.

Etxeandia, J. L. C. "La Sindone: Devozione che unisce." Second International Congress, The Shroud and Science, Turin, Italy. October 7–8, 1978.

Eusebius. *The Ecclesiastical History and the Martyrs of Palestine*. VIII:(viii):8.

Fasola, V. "Scoperte e studi archeologici dal 1939 ad oggi che concorrono ad illustrare i problemi della Santa Sindone di Torino." Second International Congress, The Shroud and Science, Turin, Italy, October 7–8, 1978.

Ferri, L., *La Sindone vista da uno sculture*. Rome: Editrice la Parola, 1978.

Feuillet, A. "L'identification et la disposition des linges tuneraines da la sepulture da Jesus d'apres les donnees do Quatrienne Evangile." Second International Congress, The Shroud and Science, Turin, Italy, October 7–8, 1978.

Feuillet, A. "The Identification and the Disposition of the Funerary Linens of Jesus' Burial According to the Data of the Fourth Gospel." *Shroud Spectrum International* 4(1982):13–23.

Filas, Francis L. "Three-Dimensional Image Analysis Confirms Pontius Pilate Coin on Shroud of Turin." *News Release* (June 11, 1981) Loyola University of Chicago.

Filas, F. J. *The Dating of the Shroud of Turin from Coins of Pontius Pilate*. Cogan Productions: Youngstown, Arizona, 1984.

Fiori, A. "Problemi e prospettive della immagini ematologiche sulla sindone." Second International Congress, The Shroud and Science, Turin, Italy, October 7–8, 1978.

Foley, C. "Carbon Dating and the Holy Shroud." *Shroud Spectrum International* 1(1982):25–27.

Fossati, L. "Copies of the Holy Shroud: Part I." *Shroud Spectrum International* 12(1986):7–23.

Fossati, L. "Copies of the Holy Shroud: Parts II and III." *Shroud Spectrum International* 13(1986):23–39.

Frean, W. *The Winding Sheet of Christ*. Ballarat, Australia, 1960.

Frei, Max. "Il passato della Sindone alla luce della palinologia." Second International Congress, The Shroud and Science, Turin, Italy, October 7–8, 1978.

Frei, M. "Nine Years of Palinological Studies on the Shroud." *Shroud Spectrum International* 3(1982):3–7.

Friend, H. *Flowers and Flower Lore.* Two vols, 1883.

Fries, T. M. *Bref och skrifvelser af och till Carl von Linne.* 1(1907):273–77.

Gadshiev, R. G., and Listengarten, A. M. *Vestnik of Dermatology and Venereology* 3(1967):86–88. Medicina, Moscow, 1967.

Garello, Edoardi. "Contributo Enigmologico su Alcune Nuove ipotesi sulla veridicita Della SS: Sindone Di Torino." In *Occasione dell' Ostensione del 1978 Collana di Enigmologia* No. 1, Edizioni 49 Flauto Magico, Torino, 1978.

Gentile, G. "Questioni d' iconografia e di cultura figurativa attorno alla Sindone." Second International Congress. The Shroud and Science, Turin, Italy. October 7–8, 1978.

Gharib, G. "La festa del Santo Mandilion nella chiesa bizantina." Second International Congress, The Shroud and Science, Turin, Italy, October 7–8, 1978.

Ghio, A. "La fotografia scientifica della Sindone." Second International Congress, The Shroud and Science, Turin, Italy, October 7–8, 1978.

Gilbert, R., Jr. and M. Marion. "Ultraviolet-Visible Reflectance and Fluorescence Spectra of the Shroud of Turin." *Applied Optics,* 19(12)(June 15, 1980):1930–1936.

Gillespie, R. et al. "Radiocarbon Measurement by Accelerator Mass Spectrometry: An Early Selection of Dates." Archaeometry 26(1984): I. 27.

Goldblatt, J. S. "The Shroud." *National Review.* (April 16, 1982):415–419.

Gonzales, T. A., M. Vance, M. Helpern and C. J. Umberger. *Legal Medicine Pathology and Toxicology.* Second ed. New York: Appleton-Century-Crofts, 1940.

Gorman, Ralph. *The Last Hours of Jesus.* New York: Sheed & Ward ed., 1960

Gove, Harry. "On Carbon-14 Dating." Unscheduled lecture at the Second International Congress, The Shroud and Science, Turin, Italy, October 7–8, 1978.

Graves, R., and J. Podro, *The Nazarene Gospel Restored.* New York: Doubleday, 1954.

Gray, H. *Anatomy of the Human Body.* Twenty-fifth ed. Edited by C. M. Goss. Philadelphia: Lea & Febiger, 1948.

Green, Maurus. "Enshrouded in Silence." *Ampleforth Journal* 74(1969).

Greig, D. M. "The Analogy of Black Colostrum to Melanhidrosis, with Some Remarks on Coloured Milk and Coloured Sweat." *Edinburgh Medical Journal,* 37(1930):524–44.

Haas, N. "Anthropological Observations on the Skeletal Remains from Giv'at ha-Mivtar." In Discoveries and Studies in Jerusalem, 1970, *Israel Exploration Journal* 20(1–2) (Jerusalem, Israel):38–59.

Haralick, R. M. *Analysis of Digital Images of the Shroud of Turin.* Monograph, private printing, Spatial Data Analysis Laboratory, Virginia Polytechnic Institute, December, 1983.

Harvey, R. C. *Some Thoughts on the Shroud of Turin.* Foundation for Christian Theology, Victoria, Texas, 1981.

Hastings, J., ed. *A Dictionary of Christ and the Gospels.* New York: Charles Scribner's Sons, 1924.

Hegi, G. *Illustrierte Flora von Mittel-Europa.* 5(1925):327–29.

Heller, John H. and Alan D. Adler. "Blood on the Shroud of Turin." *Applied Optics,* 19(16)(August 15, 1980):2742–2744.

Heller, J. H. and A. D. Adler. "A Chemical Investigation of the Turin Shroud." *Canadian Society Forensic Science Journal* 14(1981).

Heller, J. H. *Report of the Shroud of Turin.* Houghton-Mifflin. Boston, 1983.

Hengel, M. *Crucifixion in the Ancient World and the Folly of the Message of the Cross.* Fortress Press, Philadelphia, 1977.

Hersey, John. *Hiroshima.* Penguin, 1946.

Hewitt, J. W. "The Use of Nails in the Crucifixion." *Harvard Theological Review* (January 1943):29–45.

Hoare, R. *The Testimony of the Shroud.* Quartet Books, 1978.

Hoare, R. A. *Piece of Cloth, The Turin Shroud Investigated.* Aquarian Press, Ellingboro, England, 1984.

The Holy Bible, Revised Standard Version, New York: World, 1962.

Hovas, E. L. "Does the Shroud of Turin Contradict the Bible?" Personal publication, April 1984.

Humber, Thomas. *The Fifth Gospel: The Miracle of the Holy Shroud.* New York: Pocket Books, 1974.

Hurst, J. W., R. B. Loque, D. E. Rackley, R. D. Schlant, E. H. Sonnenblick, A. G. Wallace, and R. D. Wenger. *The Heart. Arteries and Veins.* Sixth Ed. New York: McGraw-Hill, 1986.

Hutchins, G. M. "Body Temperature Is Elevated in the Early Postmortem Period." *Human Pathology* 16(1985):560–561.

Hynek, R. W. *Golgotha Wissenschast and Mystik—eine medizinisch—apoligetische.* Studie uber das heilige Grablinnen von Turin, Badenia in Karlsruhe U-G. fur Berlag and Druderei, 1936.

Hynek, R. W. *Science and the Holy Shroud.* Chicago: Benedictine Press, 1936.

Hynek, R. W. *The True Likeness.* New York: Sheed & Ward, 1951.

Insinger, E. J. "A True Copy of the Shroud in Summit, New Jersey." *Shroud Spectrum International* 20(1986):25–27.

Irenueus. *Adv Haer* 2, 24, 4 Leaves used for the titulus, crux immissa.

Jackson, J. P. and E. J. Jumper. "What Space Science Detects in the Shroud." Second International Congress, Science and the Shroud, Turin, Italy, October 7–8, 1978.

Jackson, J. P., E. J. Jumper, and D. Devan. "Investigations of the Shroud of Turin by Computer Aided Analysis." *Proceedings of the 1977 United States Conference of Research on the Shroud of Turin.* (Colorado Springs, 1977):74–94.

Jackson, J. P., E. Jumper, and W. Ercoline. "Three-Dimensional Characteristics of the Shroud Image." Institute of Electric and Electronics Engineers 1982 *Proceedings of the International Conference on Cybernetics and Society,* October, 1982.

Jackson, John P., E. Jumper., and B. Mottern. (edited by Kenneth Stevenson). "The Three-Dimensional Image on Jesus' Burial Cloth." *Proceedings of the 1977 Conference of Research on the Shroud of Turin.* (Colorado Springs, 1977):190–96.

Janney, Donald H. "Computer-Aided Image Enhancement and Analysis." *Proceedings of the 1977 United States Conference of Research on the Shroud of Turin.* (Colorado Springs, 1977):146–53.

Janney, Joan. "Shroud of Turin Study. Scientists say image is that of 'Crucified' Man." Associated Press Service, October 10, 1981.

Jennings, J. A. "Putting the Shroud to Rest." *The Christian Century* 100(1983):552–554.

Johnson, C. D. "Medical and Cardiological Aspects of the Passion and Crucifixion of Jesus." *The Christ Bulletin Association Medicine.* (Puerto Rico) 70(1978):97–102.

Judica-Cordiglia, Giovanni. *L'Uomo della Sindone e il GESU del Vangeli.* Brescia: Edito dalla Fondazione P. A. Pelizza di Chiari, 1974.

Judica-Cordiglia, G. "La sepoltura di Gesu e la sacra sindone." *Salesianum* 16(1954):153–67.

Jumper, Eric J., "Considerations of Molecular Diffusion and Radiation as an Image-Formation Process on the Shroud." *Proceedings of the 1977 United States Conference of Research on the Shroud of Turin.* (Colorado Springs, 1977):182–89.

Jumper. E. J., A. D. Adler, J. P. Jackson, S. F. Pellicori, J. H. Heller, and J. R. Druzik. "A Comprehensive Examination of the Various Stains and Images on the Shroud of Turin." *Archaeological Chemistry III* No. 205(1984):447–476.

Jumper, Eric J., and Robert W. Mottern. "Scientific Investigation of the Shroud of Turin." *Applied Optics* 19(12)(June 15, 1980):1909–12.

Justinius, *The Dialogue with Trypho.* XCI, 2.

Keller, W. *The Bible as History.* New York: William Murrow & Company, 1956.

King, E. A. *Bible Plants for American Gardens.* New York: Macmillan, 1941.

Kohlbeck, J. A. and E. L. Nitowski. "New Evidence Explains Image on Shroud of Turin." *Biblical Archaeology Review* 12(1986):18–29.

Kroner, W. *Das Ratsel von Konnersreuth und Wege zu seiner Losung.* Studie eines Parapsychologen; mit einem Geleitwort. Hans Driesch, Verlag d. Aerztl. Rundschau. Munich: Otto Gmelin, 1927.

Krupp, M. A. and M. A. Chatton, *Current Medical Diagnosis and Treatment.* Los Altos, California: Lange Medical, 1978.

Krupp, M. A., M. J. Chatton and L. M. Tierney, Jr. *Current Medical Diagnosis and Treatment 1986.* Los Altos, California: Lange Medical, 1986.

Kunkle, Charles E. "Trigeminal Neuralgia." *Cecil and Loeb's Textbook of Medicine,* edited by P. Beeson and W. McDermott. Philadelphia: W. B. Saunders, 1963.

Kugelberg, E. and U. Lindblum. "The Mechanism of the Pain in Trigeminal Neuralgia." *Journal of Neurology, Neurosurgery and Psychiatry* 22(1959):26.

Lampe, Ernest W. "Surgical Anatomy of the Hand." *Clinical Symposia,* 9(1957):3–46.

Lapp, R. E. and J. R. Arnold. "Radiocarbon or Carbon-14." *World Book Encyclopedia* Q-R(1960):96.

Lavergne, C. "Gia docente agli Instituti Biblici di Gerusalemme Etude de Jean 19:25 a 20:18." Second International Congress, The Shroud and Science, Turin, Italy, October 7–8, 1978.

Lavoie, B. B., G. R. Lavoie, D. Klutstein, and J. Regan. "In Accordance with Jewish Burial Custom, the Body of Jesus was not Washed." *Sindon* 30(1981). Turin, Italy.

Lavoie, G. R., B. B. Lavoie and A. D. Adler. "Blood on the Shroud of Turin: Part III. The Blood on the Face." *Shroud Spectrum International* 20(1986):3–16.

Lavoie, G. R., B. B. Lavoie, V. J. Donovan, and J. S. Ballas. "Blood on the Shroud of Turin: Part II." *Shroud Spectrum International* 8(1983):2–8.

Lavsky, G. K. (Hematidrosis), Soviet Clinic 1(1932) p. 48.

LeBec, A. A. "Physiological Study of the Passion of Our Lord Jesus Christ." *The Catholic Medical Guardian* 3:126 1925.

LeBec, A. "Le Supplice de la Croix." *L'Evangile dans la vie* April, 1925

Levi-Setti, R., G. Crow, and Y. L. Wano. "Progress in High Resolution Scanning Ion Microscopy and Secondary Ion Mass Spectrometry Imaging Microanalysis." *Scanning Electron Microscopy* 2(1985):535–551.

Lidell-Scott. *Greek-English Lexicon.* Seventh Ed. New York: Harper Brothers, 1883.

Lipsius, Justus. *De Cruce. Libri tres, ad sacram profanamque historiam utiles.* (3d part, Tome III, *Opera Omnia* Antwerp, 1614).

Livy. *Liber XXXIII, 36.*

Lorre, J. J., and D. J. Lynn. "Digital Enhancement of Images of the Shroud of Turin." *Proceedings of the 1977 United States Conference of Research on the Shroud of Turin.* (Colorado Springs, 1977):154–81.

Lovie, J. "La Saint-Suarie en Savoie." Second International Congress, The Shroud and Science, Turin, Italy, October 7–8, 1978.

Lucanus. *Pharsalia.* Lib. Vi, 547.

Lumpkin, R. "The Physical Suffering of Christ." *Journal of the Medical Association of the State of Alabama* 47(1978):8–10, 47.

Marfan, A. B. "Un Cas de deformation congenitale des quatre membres plus prononcee aux extremites characterisee par l'allongement des os avec un certain degre d'amini cessement." *Bulletin Memorial Society Medicine Hospital* Paris, 13(1896):220.

Mayer, J. K. "Die Erkrankungen der Schweissdrusen." In *Jadassohn Handb. d. Haut-u. Geschlechtskr.* Vol. 13. Berlin: J. Springer, 1932.

McCown, T. M. "Cloth-Body Distance of the Holy Shroud." *Proceedings of the 1977 United States Conference of Research on the Shroud of Turin.* (Colorado Springs, 1977):95–109.

McCrone, Walter C. "Authentication of the Turin Shroud." *Proceedings of the 1977 United States Conference of Research on the Shroud of Turin.* (Colorado Springs, 1977):124–30.

McCrone, Walter C. and Christine Skirius. "Light Microscopical Study of the Turin 'Shroud' I." Reprinted from *The Microscope* 28(3/4)1980.

McCrone, W. C., "Light Microscopical Study of the Turin 'Shroud' II." Reprinted from *The Microscope* 28(3/4)1980.

McCrone, W. C. "What We Found on the Turin Shroud and How We Found It." *Functional Photography* 16(3, May/June 1981):19, 20, 30.

McCrone, W. C. "Current Look at Carbon Dating." *La Sindone e la Scienza.* Turin, Italy, 1978.

McCrone, W. C. "Shroud Image Is the Work of an Artist." *The Skeptical Inquirer.* 6(1986):35–36.

McEvoy, W. *The Death Image of Christ.* Melbourne, Australia, 1945.

McKusick, V. A. "Marfan's Syndrome." In *The Metabolic Basis of Inherited Disease.* Edited by J. B. Stanbury, J. B. Wyngaarden, and D. S. Frederickson, pp. 1381–1382. New York: McGraw-Hill, 1978.

McKusick, V. A. *Heritable Disorders of Connective Tissue.* Fourth ed. St. Louis: Mosby. 1972.

Meacham, H. "The Authentication of the Turin Shroud: An Issue in Archaeological Epistemology." *Current Anthropology* 24(1983):282–311.

Meacham, W. "On Carbon Dating the Turin Shroud." *Shroud Spectrum International* 19(1986):15–25.

Meyer, Karl E. "Were You There When They Photographed My Lord?" *Esquire* (August) 1971.

Mikulicz-Radeki, F. V. "The Chest Wound in the Crucified Christ." *Medical News.* 14(1966):30–40.

Miller, V. C., and S. F. Pellicori. "Ultraviolet Fluorescence Photography of the Shroud of Turin." *Journal of Biological Photography,* 49(3)(July 1981):71–85.

Mills, A. A. "A Corona-Discharge Hypothesis for the Mechanism of Image Formation on the Turin Shroud." Proceedings of the British Society for the Turin Shroud. Autumn 1979. Summer 1981.

Moedder, H. *Die Todersursache Bei der Kreuzigung: Stimmer der Zeit.* March, 1949.

Moldenke, H. N. and A. L. Moldenke. *Plants of the Bible.* New York: Ronald Press, 1952.

Mole, R. H. "Fibrinolysin and Fluidity of Blood Post Mortem." *Journal of Pathology and Bacteriology,* 60(1948):430.

Monheim, L. M. "Local Anesthesia and Pain Control." In *Dental Practice,* C. V. Mosby Co., St. Louis. Second Ed., 1961.

Morano, E. "Aspetti ultrastrutturali al Microscopio ellectronico a scansion e di fibre della Sindone." Second International Congress, The Shroud and Science, Turin, Italy, October 7–8, 1978.

Morgan, R., *Perpetual Miracle.* Runciman Press, Manly, Australia, 1980.

Morgan, R. *Shroud Guide.* Runciman Press, Manly, Australia, 1983.

Morgan, R. *The Holy Shroud and the Earliest Paintings of Christ.* Runciman Press, Manly, Australia, 1986.

Mueller, M. M. "The Shroud of Turin: A Critical Appraisal." *The Skeptical Inquirer* 6(1986)15–33.

Murdock, J. L., B. A. Walker, B. L. Halpern, J. A. Kuzma, and V. A. McKusick. "Life Expectancy and Causes of Death in the Marfan Syndrome." *New England Journal of Medicine* 286(1972):804.

Murphy, C. "Shreds of Evidence." *Harper's* (November, 1981):42–65.

Naclerio, E. A. *Chest Injuries, Physiological Principles and Emergency Management.* New York: Grune & Stratton, 1971.

Naveh, J. "The Ossuary Inscriptions from Giv'at ha-Mivtar." *Israel Exploration Journal* 20(1970):33–37.

Nickell, Joe. "The Turin Shroud: Fake? Fact? Photograph?" *Popular Photography* 85 November (1979):97–99, 146, 147.

Nickell, Joe. "New Evidence: The Shroud of Turin Is a Forgery." *Free Inquiry* (Summer 1981):28–30.

Nickell, J. "The Shroud of Turin—Solved! *The Humanist* 38(1978):30–32.

Nickell, J. *Inquest on the Shroud of Turin.* Prometheus Books: Buffalo, 1983.

"Numismatic Error Confirms Shroud's Coin." Editorial, *World Coin News,* September 22, 1981.

O'Connell, P., and C. Carty, *The Holy Shroud and Four Visions.* Tan Books: Rockford, Il, 1974.

O'Gorman, P. W. "The Holy Shroud of Jesus Christ: New Discovery of the Cause of the Impression." *American Ecclesiastical Review,* vol. 102, 1940.

O'Rahilly, A., "The Burial of Christ." *Irish Ecclesiastical Record,* vol. 59, 1941.

O'Rahilly, A. *The Crucified.* (Edited by J. A. Gaughan) Kingdom Books: Dublin, 1985.

Orchard D. B., E. F. Sutcliffe, R. C. Fuller, and D. R. Russell. *A Catholic Commentary on Holy Scripture*. New York: Thomas Nelson & Sons, 1953.

Otterbein, Adam. "The Holy Shroud." *The New Catholic Encyclopedia*. Vol. 13. New York, 1967.

Otterbein, Adam. "Introduction to the Shroud and State of the Question." *Proceedings of the 1977 United States Conference of Research on the Shroud of Turin*. (Colorado Springs, 1977):1–9.

Pellicori, S. F., and R. A. Chandos. "Portable Unit Permits UV/Vis Study of 'Shroud'." Reprinted from *Industrial Research & Development*, February, 1981.

Pellicori, Samuel, with Mark S. Evans. "The Shroud of Turin Through the Microscope." *Archaeology*. (January/February 1981):34–43.

"Photograph of the Holy Shroud by Electric Light" (from report appearing in August 6, 1898 issue of *Scientific American*).

Pia, S. "Memoria sulla riproduzione fotografica de la santissima Sindone. (original 1902). Published in *Sindon*, 1960.

Pia, S. Letter to Dr. Cavaliere Benedetto Porro, February 28, 1901. Turin, Italy. *Shroud Spectrum International* 18(1986):7–11.

Pickl. "Messiaskoenig Jesus." In *der Auffassung seiner Zeitgenossen* pp. 156–63. Munich: Koesel-Pustet, 1935.

Plutarch, *Moralia*. *De sera numinis vindicata*. IX.

Polybius. *The Histories*, Liber 1, 86.

Post, G. E. *Flora of Syria, Palestine, and Sinai*. Vol. 11, 1933.

Pozzo, A. "Cromidrosi rossa ascellare legata a iniezioni di jodo bismutato di chinino." *Giornale veneto di scienze medica*, 8(1934):486–89.

Primrose, W. B. "A Surgeon Looks at the Crucifixion." *The Hibbert Journal*, 47(1949):382–88.

Raes, G. "Rapport d'Analyse du Tissu." *La S. Sindone Richerche e Studi della Commissione di Esperti nominati dall Archivescovo di Torino, nel poe* 79–85, 1969, 1976.

Reban, John (Hans Naber). *Inquest on Jesus Christ—Did He Die on the Cross?* London: Leslie Frewin, 1967.

Rentoul, E., and H. Smith. *Glaister's Medical Jurisprudence and Toxicology*. Thirteenth ed. (pp. 155–63) Edinburgh and London: Churchill Livingstone, 1973.

Report of the Turin Commission on The Holy Shroud. London, 1976.

Rhein, R. W., Jr. "The Shroud of Turin." *Medical World News*, (McGraw-Hill Publication) 20(1980):40–50.

Ricci, G. "Evangelizzazione e Santa Sindone." Second International Congress, The Shroud and Science, Turin, Italy, October 7–8, 1978.

Ricci, G. "Historical, Medical and Physical Study of the Holy Shroud." *Proceedings of the 1977 United States Conference of Research on the Shroud of Turin*. (Colorado Springs, 1977):58–73.

Ricci, G. *L'Uomo della sindone e Gesu*. Rome, 1969.

Ricciotti, G. *The Life of Christ*. Translated by Alba I. Zizzamia. Milwaukee: Bruce, 1947.

Riecke, E. "Hematidrosis," in *Lehrbuch der Haut und Gesechkechtskrankheiten* (p. 310) Jena, 1923.

Rinaldi, Peter. "A Summary of the Critique of the Report of the Turin Commission on the Holy Shroud." *Proceedings of the United States Conference of Research on the Shroud of Turin*. (Colorado Springs, 1977):58–73.

Rinaldi, Peter M. "The Holy Shroud." *Sign* XIII (June 1934):685–688.

Rinaldi, Peter M. "I Saw the Holy Shroud." *Sign* LIII, (February 1974).

Rinaldi, Peter M. *I Saw the Holy Shroud.* Tampa, Florida: Don Bosco Messenger, 1938.

Rinaldi, Peter M. *It Is the Lord.* New York: Vantage Press, 1972.

Rinaldi, P. M., *When Missions Saw the Shroud.* New Rochelle: Don Bosco, 1979.

Rinaldi, P. M., "On Disproving the Shroud of Turin." (A rebuttal to articles in *Skeptical Inquirer.*) 3(1982):15–56, ("Special Critique on the Shroud of Turin").

Robbins, S. L. *Pathologic Basis of Disease.* Philadelphia: W. B. Saunders, 1974.

Robbins, S. L. and R. S. Cotran. *Pathologic Basis of Disease.* Second Ed. Philadelphia: W. B. Saunders, 1979.

Robbins, S. L., R. S. Cotran, and V. Kumar. *Pathologic Basis of Disease.* Third Ed. Philadelphia: W. B. Saunders, 1984.

Robinson, John. "The Shroud and the New Testament." Second International Congress, The Shroud and Science, Turin, Italy, October 7–8, 1978.

Robinson, John A. T. "The Shroud of Turin and the Grave Cloths of the Gospels." *Proceedings of the United States Conference of Research on the Shroud of Turin.* (Colorado Springs, 1977):23–30.

Rodante, S. "La Sindone: Testimonianza della morte vera d. Cristo." Second International Congress, The Shroud and Science, Turin, Italy, October 7–8, 1978.

Rogers, Ray N. "Chemical Considerations Concerning the Shroud of Turin." *Proceedings of the 1977 United States Conference of Research on the Shroud of Turin.* (Colorado Springs, 1977):131–35.

Rosomoff, H. L. and F. T. Zugibe. "Distribution of the Intracranial Contents in Experimental Edema." *Archives Neurology,* 9(1963):26–34.

Roth, H. L. *Ancient Egyptian and Greek Looms.* Bankfield Museum: Halifax, 1974.

Rothman, S. and F. Schaaf. "Chemie der Haut." In *Jadassohn, Handb. d. Haut-u. Geschlechtskr* 1/2(1929):161–377. Berlin: J. Springer.

Rothman, Stephen. *Physiology and Biochemistry of the Skin.* Chicago: University of Chicago Press, 1954.

Ruark, H. C. "The Continuing Search . . . New Findings Focus on Shroud of Turin." *Functional Photography.* 16(3)(May/June 1981):18, 30–39.

Salvi, B. M. M. "Revisione critica anatomica sulle lesioni della mano e del polso dell' Llomo della Sindone." Second International Congress, The Shroud and Science, Turin, Italy, October 7–8, 1978.

Samberger, F. "Chromidrosis." *Dermat, Wchnschr* 109(1939):806–812, 1939.

Sammaccia, B. and A. E. Burakowski. *The Eucharistic Miracle of Lanciano.* Kuba: Trumbull, CT, 1976.

Sandhurt, B. G. "The Silent Witness." Unpublished manuscript from the collection of Rev. Maurus Green, O.S.B.

Sava, Anthony. "The Blood and Water from the Side of Christ." *American Ecclesiastical Review* 138(1958):341–45.

Savio, P. "The Arrangement of the Sindon when It Unfolded the Body of Christ." *Shroud Spectrum International* 12(1986):24–27.

Schafersman, S. D. "Science, the Public and the Shroud of Turin." *The Skeptical Inquirer* 6(1986)37–55.

Schwalbe, L. A. and R. N. Robers. "Physics and Chemistry of Shroud of Turin—A Summary of the 1978 Investigation." *Analytica Chimica Acta* 135(1982):3–49.

Schwerin, F., Grav von. "Kreuzeholz und Dornenkrone." In *Mitteilungen der Deutsche Dendrologische Gesellschaft* 45(1933):155–57.

Scott, C. T. "A Case of Hematidrosis." *British Medical Journal,* May 11, 1918.

Seneca. *Ad Lucilius Epistulae morales.* Epistle Cl.

Seneca. *Moral Essays,* III, I.

Shelley. W. B. and H. J. Hurley. "Methods of Exploring Human Apocrine Sweat Gland Physiology." *Archives Dermatology and Syphololology,* 6(1952):156–61.

Shelley, W. B. and H. Hurley. "The Physiology of the Human Axillary Apocrine Sweat Gland." *Archives Dermatology and Syphololology* 20(1953):285–97.

Shroud of Turin Research Project. Symposium of Research Findings, Connecticut College, New London, Connecticut, October 10 and 11, 1981.

Simpson, K. *Forensic Medicine.* London: Edward Arnold Publishers, Ltd., 1964.

Skinner, C. M. *Myths and Legends of Flowers, Trees, Fruits and Plants in All Ages and All Climes.* received in Journal of Botany (British and Foreign) 64:(1926).

Smith, J. *Bible Plants, Their History, with a Review of the Opinions of Various Writers Regarding Their Identification.* 1878.

Smith, W., ed. *A Dictionary of the Bible, Comprising Its Antiquities, Biography, Geography and Natural History.* 1876.

Snedecor, S. T. "The Crucifixion—In the Eyes of a Physician." *Reformed Church Review—Senusures of Reformed Church in America.* (April 1973):189–94.

Sorgia, R. "La Sindone prova della morte e teste della Resurrezione di Cristo." Second International Congress, The Shroud and Science, Turin, Italy, October 7–8, 1978.

Sox, H. D. "Bringing the Shroud to the Test," in *Face to Face with the Turin Shroud.* Oxford, 1978.

Sox, H. D. *File on the Shroud.* Coronet Books, 1978.

Sox, H. D. *The Image on the Shroud. Is the Turin Shroud a Forgery?* Unwin Publications, 1981.

Spinner, Morton. *Injuries to the Major Branches of Peripheral Nerves of the Forearm.* Second ed. Philadelphia: W. B. Saunders, 1978.

Spitz, W. U. and R. S. Fisher. *Medicolegal Investigation of Death.* Springfield, Illinois: Charles C. Thomas, 1973 and 1980.

Stevenson, K. E., and G. R. Habermas. *Verdict on the Shroud.* Servant Books: Ann Arbor, Michigan, 1981.

Stimpson, G. W. *Popular Questions Answered.* George Sully and Company, Inc., 1931.

Stroud, W. *A Treatise on the Physical Cause of the Death of Christ.* London: Hamilton & Adams, 1874.

Sullivan, Barbara M. "How in Fact Was Jesus Lain in the Tomb?" *National Review,* July 20, 1973.

Swan, G., and L. Sodeman. *Pathological Physiology.* Fourth ed. Philadelphia: W. B. Saunders, 1967.

Szodoray, L. "Heterotopic apocrine glands." *Orvosi hetil.* 4(1948):360, Quoted in *Excerpta med.* Sec. XIII, 3(1949):382.

Tamburelli, G. "The Shroud as Seen by Computer." *La Sindone* supplementide La Stampa, Torino, 27 Agosto–8 Ottobre 1978.

Tamburelli, G. "Riceca dell' impronta dell' ombelico nell' immagine Sindonica." *La Sindone* 29(December 1980):33–37.

Tamburelli, G. "Some Results in the Processing of the Holy Shroud of Turin." Institute of Electric and Electronic Engineers Transaction on Pattern Analysis and Machine Intelligence PAMI-3 (6)(November 1981):17–24.

Tamburelli, G. Studio della Sindone mediante il calcolatore elettronico. *L'Elettrotechnica* (12)70:1983.

Tamburelli, G. Impronta Sindonica Della Monetina Rivelvata Dal Computer Sindone, 1984.

Tamburelli, G. "An Image Resurrection of the Man on the Shroud." *Shroud Spectrum International* 15(1985):3–6.

Tamburelli, G., and G. Garoboto. "Nuovi syiluppi nell' elaborazione della immagine Sindonica." Second International Congress, The Shroud and Science, Turin, Italy, October 7–8, 1978.

Tedeschi, Eckert, and Cesare Tedeschi. *Forensic Medicine: A Study in Trauma and Environmental Hazards.* Vols 1–3, Philadelphia: W. B. Saunders, 1977.

Tenney, S. M. "On Death by Crucifixion." *American Heart Journal* 68(1964):286–287.

Terrien, S. "The Clown at the King's Game." Lecture in Atlantic City, New Jersey, March 26, 1981.

"The Lost Gospel According to Peter," in *The Lost Books of the Bible and the Forgotten Books of Eden.* Fount Religious Prayerbook Series, Collins Publications, Cleveland, 1948.

Thomas, M. "The Shroud of Turin." *Rolling Stone* December 27, 1978–January 11, 1979.

Thurston, Herbert. "The Holy Shroud as a Scientific Problem." *The Month*, Vol. CI, 1903.

Tribbe, F. *Portrait of Jesus.* New York: Stein and Day, 1983.

Tyrer, J. "Notes upon the Turin Shroud as a Textile." *General Report and Proceedings of the British Society for the Turin Shroud* (Autumn 1979, Summer 1971).

Tyrer, J. "Looking at the Turin Shroud as a Textile." *Shroud Spectrum International* 6(1983):35–45.

Tzaferis, V. "Jewish Tombs at and near Giv' at ha Mivtar." *Jerusalem Israel Exploration Journal,* 20(1970):18–32.

Tzaferis, V. "Crucifixion, The Archaeological Evidence." *Biblical Archaeology Review* 11(1985):44–53.

Vignon, P. *Le Saint Suaire De Turin, devant la Science, l'archeologie, l'histoire, l'iconographie la logique.* Paris: Masson et Cie; Editeuri Saint Germaine, Blvd., 1938.

Vignon, P. *The Shroud of Christ.* New Hyde Part, New York: University Books, 1970.

Vignon, P. and Edward Wuenschel. "The Problem of the Holy Shroud." *Scientific American* 93(1937):162–64.

Volckringer, J. *Le Probleme des empreintes devant de la science.* Paris Libraire de Carmel, 1942.

Wacks, M. "Shroud of Turin Numismatic Controversy, *The Augur.*" *Journal of Biblical Numismatic Society* 35(1982):137.

Walsh, John. *The Shroud.* New York: Random House, 1963.

Wassenar, R. A. "Physician Looks at the Suffering Christ." *Moody* (March 1979):41–42.

Weaver, K. "The Mystery of the Shroud." *National Geographic* 157:730–753, June 1980.

Webb, C. "Scientific Photography and the Shroud of Turin." *Proceedings of the United States Conference of Research on the Shroud of Turin.* (Colorado Springs, 1977).

Wedenisson, U. "Considerazioni ipotetiche sulla cause fiscia della morte dell' llomo della sindone." Second International Congress. The Shroud and Science, Turin, Italy, October 7–8, 1978.

Weyland, P. "Some Problems Connected with Crucifixion." (Lectures).

Weyland, Peter. *A Sculptor Interprets the Holy Shroud of Turin.* Esopus, New York: The Holy Shroud Guild, 1954.

Whanger, A., and M. Whanger. "Polarized Image Overlay Technique: A New Image Comparison Method and Its Applications." *Applied Optics* 24(1985):766–772.

White, J., and W. Sweet. "Facial and Cephalic Neuralgias: Trigeminal neuralgia" (Tic Douloureux, Trifacial Neuralgia). *Pain: Its Mechanism and Neurosurgical Control,* Charles C. Thomas Publishers, Springfield, Ohio, pp. 433–37, 1955.

Wilcox, R. L. *Shroud.* New York: Macmillan, 1977.

Wild, R. A. "The Shroud of Turin. Probably the work of a 14th Century Artist or Forger." *Biblical Archaeology Review* 10(1984):30–46.

Willis, David. "Did He Die on the Cross?" *Ampleforth Journal,* vol. 74, 1969.

Wilson, Ian. "A Gift to Our Proof-demanding Era?" *Catholic Herald* (London), November 16, 1973.

Wilson, Ian. "New Insights in the History of the Holy Shroud." Second International Congress, The Shroud and Science, Turin, Italy, October 7–8, 1978.

Wilson, Ian. *The Shroud of Turin, the Burial Cloth of Jesus Christ?* Garden City, New York: Lange Books, 1979.

Wilson, I. and V. Miller. *The Mysterious Shroud.* Doubleday: New York, 1986.

Wuenschel, Edward A. "The Photograph of Christ." *Parx* 15(1937):112–15.

Wuenschel, Edward A. "The Holy Shroud: Present State of the Question." *American Ecclesiastical Review* 102(1940):465–86.

Yudin, S. S. *Lancet,* 2:361, 1937.

Zeuli, T., and B. Barberis. "La Sindone e la scienza." *Lions Club Rivol,* Valsasa, 1978.

Zias, J., and E. Sekeles. "The Crucified Man from Giv' at ha-Mivtar." *Israel Exploration Journal* 35(1985):22–27.

Zimmerman, M. R. "Blood Cells Preserved in a Mummy 2000 Years Old." *Science* 180(1973): 303–304.

Zohary, M., "The Arboreal Flora of Israel and Transjordan and Its Ecological and Phytogeographical Significance." In Imperial Forestry Institute, University of Oxford, *Institute Paper* 26, 1951.

Zorell, F. *Lexicon Hebraicum et Aramaicum Veters Testamenti,* 7 Fascicles, Biblical Institute Press, Rome, 1950.

Zugibe, F. T. "Our Crucified God." *Tertiary Topics, Third Order of St. Francis,* 14(March 1961):1–4.

Zugibe, F. T. *Eat, Drink and Lower Your Cholesterol.* New York. McGraw-Hill, 1963.

Zugibe, F. T. "Histochemical Studies in Coronary Atherogenesis: Comparison with Aortic and Cerebral Atherogenesis." *Circulation Research* 3(1963)401–9.

Zugibe, F. T. "Relationship between Chondroitin Sulfate Collagen in Atherosclerosis." *Proceedings of International Congress on Atherogenesis, Paris.* Edited by L. Scebat, Publisher, Spring, 1968. Le Role de la paroi arterielle dans la atherogenese colloques Internationaux due Centre Nationale de la Recherche Scientifique. No. 129, Paris 1967, Centre National de le Recherche Scientifique.

Zugibe, F. T. *Diagnostic Histochemistry.* St. Louis: Mosby, 1970.

Zugibe, F. T. *The Cross and the Shroud. A Medical Examiner Investigates the Crucifixion.* Angelus Books: Garnerville, New York, 1982.

Zugibe, F. T. *Death by Crucifixion.* Canadian Society Forensic Science Journal 17(1983):1–13.

Zugibe, F. T. "Death by Crucifixion, Queries and Commments." *Biblical Archaeology Review* 11(1985):24.

Zugibe, F. T., "Still More on the Shroud: Queries and Comments." *Biblical Archaeology Review* 13 (1987): 63–65.

Zugibe, F. T. "The Crucifixion of Jesus: Areas of Controversy." *Biblical Archaeology Review.* (In press).

Zugibe, F. T. "Did Jesus Die of Marfan's Disease?" *Medical Heritage.* (In press).

Zugibe, F. T., P. Bell, Jr., and T. Conley. "Radiopaque Plastic Injection Technique for Assessing Coronary Stenosis and Collateralization at Autopsy." *Circulation,* 29:32–33, 1964.

Zugibe, F. T. and K. D. Brown. "Histochemistry of the Cerebral Arteries." *Circulation* 20(1959):971.

Zugibe, F. T. and K. D. Brown. "Histochemical Studies of Atherogenesis: Human Aortas." *Circulation Research* 8(1960):287.

Zugibe, F. T. and K. D. Brown. "Histochemistry of the Coronary Arteries." *Circulation* 21(1960):654.

Zugibe, F. T. and K. D. Brown. "Histochemical Studies in Atherogenesis: Human Cerebral Arteries." *Circulation Research* 9(1961):897–905.

Zugibe, F. T., T. Conley, and P. Bell, Jr. "Grading Coronary Stenosing." *Circulation* 29(1964):33.

Zugibe, F. T., T. Conley, P. Bell, Jr., and M. Standish. "Assessing Myocardial Alterations at Autopsy in the Absence of Gross and Microscopic Changes." *Circulation* 37(1965):218.

Zugibe, F. T., T. Conley, P. Bell, Jr., and M. Standish. "Determination of Myocardial Alterations at Autopsy in the Absence of Gross and Microscopic Changes." *Archives Pathology* 81(1966):409.

Zugibe, F. T., T. Conley, P. Bell, Jr.,and M. Standish. "Enzyme Decay Curves in Normal and Infarcted Myocardium." *Archives Pathology* 93(1972):308, 311.

Index

NOTE: Boldface page numbers indicate illustrations.

229